High-Yield™

Embryology

FIFTH EDITION

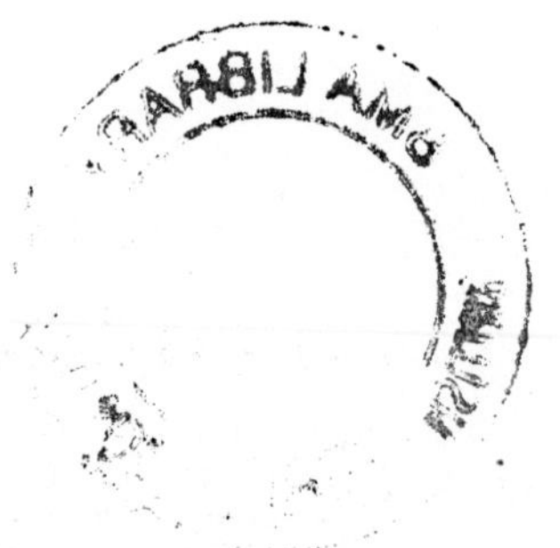

High-Yield™

Embryology

FIFTH EDITION

Ronald W. Dudek, PhD
Professor
Brody School of Medicine
East Carolina University
Department of Anatomy and Cell Biology
Greenville, North Carolina

Wolters Kluwer | Lippincott Williams & Wilkins
Health
Philadelphia • Baltimore • New York • London
Buenos Aires • Hong Kong • Sydney • Tokyo

Acquisitions Editor: Crystal Taylor
Product Manager: Lauren Pecarich
Marketing Manager: Joy Fisher Williams
Vendor Manager: Bridgett Dougherty
Manufacturing Manager: Margie Orzech
Design Coordinator: Terry Mallon
Compositor: S4Carlisle Publishing Services

351 West Camden Street
Baltimore, MD 21201

530 Walnut Street
Philadelphia, PA 19106

Printed in China

9 8 7 6 5 4 3 2 1

Library of Congress Cataloging-in-Publication Data

ISBN-13: 978-1-4511-7610-0
ISBN-10: 1-4511-7610-4

Cataloging-in-Publication data available on request from the Publisher.

To purchase additional copies of this book, call our customer service department at **(800) 638-3030** or fax orders to **(301) 223-2320**. International customers should call **(301) 223-2300**.

Visit Lippincott Williams & Wilkins on the Internet: http://www.lww.com. Lippincott Williams & Wilkins customer service representatives are available from 8:30 am to 6:00 pm, EST.

CCS0413

I would like to dedicate this book to
my father, Stanley J. Dudek, who died
Sunday, March 20, 1988, at 11 A.M.
It was his hard work and sacrifice
that allowed me access to the finest
educational institutions in the country
(St. John's University in Collegeville, MN;
the University of Minnesota Medical School;
Northwestern University; and the University
of Chicago). It was by hard work and
sacrifice that he showed his love for his wife,
Lottie; daughter, Christine; and grandchildren,
Karolyn, Katie, and Jeannie.
I remember my father often as a good man
who did the best he could.
Who could ask for more?
My father is missed and remembered by many.

Preface

The fifth edition of *High-Yield™ Embryology* includes improvements based on suggestions and comments from the many medical students who have used this book in preparation for the USMLE Step 1 examination and those students who have reviewed the book. I pay close attention to these suggestions and comments in order to improve the quality of this book. The goal of *High-Yield™ Embryology* is to provide an accurate and quick review of important clinical aspects of embryology for the future physician.

Many times in the history of science, certain biological concepts become entrenched and accepted as dogma even though recent evidence comes to light to challenge these concepts. One of these concepts is the process of twinning. Recent evidence calls into question the standard figures used in textbooks on how the process of twinning occurs. In particular, it is becoming increasingly difficult to ignore the fact that dizygotic twins are sometimes monochorionic. Although we by far do not know or attempt to explain exactly how twinning occurs, it seems that the interesting cell and molecular events involved in twinning occur in the first few cell divisions during first three or four days after fertilization. You are not a twin because the inner cell mass splits. The inner cell mass splits because you are a twin. This evidence warrants a new twinning figure (Figure 2-2) that does not comport with the standard figures but tries to embrace recent evidence although many may call it controversial. Progress in our scientific understanding of twinning will never occur if our concept of the twinning process is overly simplistic and reinforced by standard figures repeated over and over in textbooks. Some published references that speak to this twinning issue include Boklage (2009, 2010), Yoon et al. (2005), Williams et al. (2004), and Hoekstra et al. (2008).

I understand that *High-Yield™ Embryology* is a review book designed for a USMLE Step 1 review and that you will not be faced with a question regarding this twinning concept, but I know my readers are sophisticated enough to appreciate the scientific and clinical value of being challenged to question traditional concepts as "grist for the mill" in discussions with your colleagues.

I would appreciate receiving your comments and/or suggestions concerning *High-Yield™ Embryology*, Fifth Edition, especially after you have taken the USMLE Step 1 examination. Your suggestions will find their way into the sixth edition. You may contact me at dudekr@ecu.edu.

References

Boklage CE. Traces of embryogenesis are the same in monozygotic and dizygotic twins: not compatible with double ovulation. *Hum Reprod.* 2009;24(6):1255–1266.

Boklage CE. *How New Humans Are Made: Cells and Embryos, Twins and Chimeras, Left and Right, Mind/Self/Soul, Sex, and Schizophrenia.* Hackensack, NJ; London: World Scientific Publishing; 2010.

Yoon G, Beischel LS, Johnson JP, et al. Dizygotic twin pregnancy conceived with assisted reproductive technology associated with chromosomal anomaly, imprinting disorder, and monochorionic placentation. *J Pediatr.* 2005;146:565–567.

Williams CA, Wallace MR, Drury KC, et al. Blood lymphocyte chimerism associated with IVF and monochorionic dizygous twinning: Case report. *Hum Reprod.* 2004;19(12):2816–2821.

Hoekstra C, Zhao ZZ, Lambalk CB, et al. Dizygotic twinning. *Hum Reprod Update.* 2008;14(1):37–47.

Contents

Chapter **1**

Prefertilization Events

I Gametes (Oocytes and Spermatozoa)

A. Are descendants of **primordial germ cells** that originate in the wall of the yolk sac of the embryo and migrate into the gonad region.

B. Are produced in the adult by either **oogenesis** or **spermatogenesis**, processes that involve **meiosis.**

II Meiosis

A. Occurs **only during the production of gametes.**

B. Consists of two cell divisions (**meiosis I and meiosis II**) and results in the formation of gametes containing 23 chromosomes and 1N amount of DNA (23,1N).

C. Promotes the exchange of small amounts of maternal and paternal DNA via **crossover** during meiosis I.

III Female Gametogenesis (Oogenesis) (Figure 1-1)

A. **PRIMORDIAL GERM CELLS (46,2N)** from the wall of the yolk sac arrive in the ovary at week 6 of embryonic development and differentiate into **oogonia** (46,2N).

B. Oogonia enter **meiosis I** and undergo DNA replication to form **primary oocytes** (46,4N). All primary oocytes are formed by the **fifth month of fetal life** and remain dormant in **prophase (dictyotene stage) of meiosis I until puberty**.

C. During a woman's ovarian cycle, a primary oocyte completes meiosis I to form a **secondary oocyte** (23,2N) and a **first polar body**, which probably degenerates.

D. The secondary oocyte enters **meiosis II**, and ovulation occurs when the chromosomes align at metaphase. The secondary oocyte remains **arrested in metaphase of meiosis II** until fertilization occurs.

E. At fertilization, the secondary oocyte completes meiosis II to form a **mature oocyte** (23,1N) and a **second polar body**.

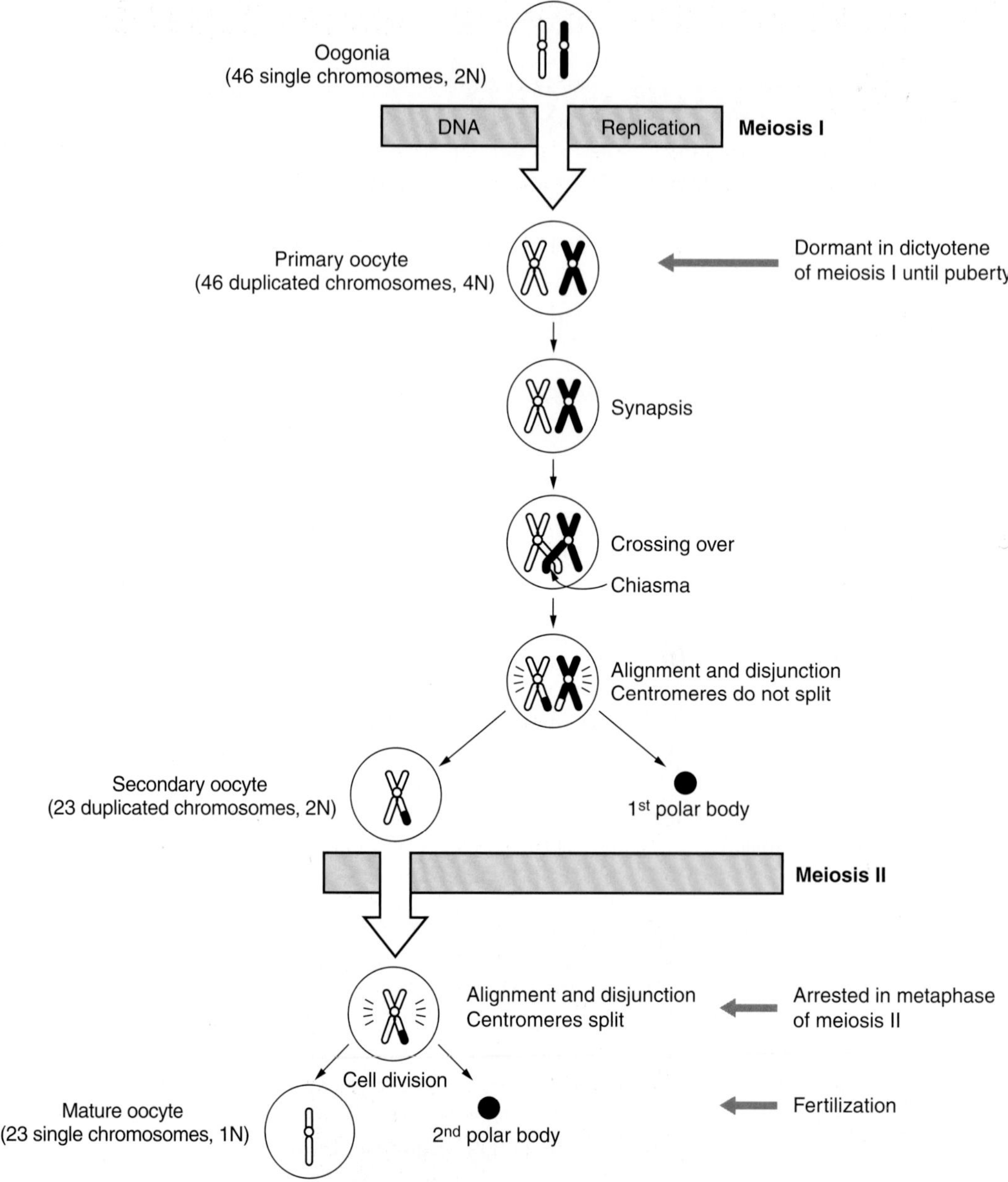

● **Figure 1-1 Female gametogenesis (oogenesis).** Note that only one pair of homologous chromosomes is shown (white = maternal origin; black = paternal origin). Synapsis is the process of pairing of homologous chromosomes. The point at which the DNA molecule crosses over is called the chiasma and is where exchange of small amounts of maternal and paternal DNA occurs. Note that synapsis and crossing over occur only during meiosis I. The polar bodies are storage bodies for DNA unnecessary for the further function of the cell and probably degenerate. There is no evidence that polar bodies divide or undergo any other activity.

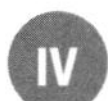

IV Hormonal Control of the Female Reproductive Cycle (Figure 1-2)

A. The hypothalamus secretes **gonadotropin-releasing factor (GnRF).**

B. In response to GnRH, the adenohypophysis secretes the gonadotropins, **follicle-stimulating hormone (FSH) and luteinizing hormone (LH).**

C. FSH stimulates the development of a secondary follicle to a Graafian follicle within the ovary.

D. Granulosa cells of the secondary and Graafian follicle secrete **estrogen.**

E. Estrogen stimulates the endometrium of the uterus to enter the proliferative phase.

F. LH stimulates ovulation.

G. Following ovulation, granulosa lutein cells of the corpus luteum secrete **progesterone.**

H. Progesterone stimulates the endometrium of the uterus to enter the secretory phase.

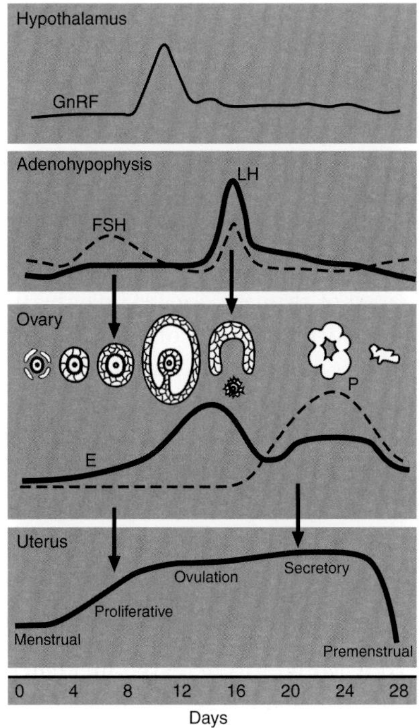

● **Figure 1-2 Hormonal control of the female reproductive cycle.** The various patterns of hormone secretion from the hypothalamus, adenohypophysis, and ovary are shown. These hormones prepare the endometrium of the uterus for implantation of a conceptus. The menstrual cycle of the uterus includes the following: (1) The menstrual phase (days 1–4), which is characterized by the **necrosis and shedding** of the functional layer of the endometrium. (2) The proliferative phase (days 4–15), which is characterized by the **regeneration** of the functional layer of the endometrium and a **low basal body temperature** (97.5°F). (3) The ovulatory phase (14–16), which is characterized by **ovulation** of a secondary oocyte and coincides with the LH surge. (4) The secretory phase (days 15–25), which is characterized by **secretory activity** of the endometrial glands and an **elevated basal body temperature** (98°F). Implantation of a conceptus occurs in this phase. (5) Premenstrual phase (days 25–28), which is characterized by **ischemia** due to reduced blood flow to the endometrium. E = estrogen; FSH = follicle-stimulating hormone; GnRF = gonadotropin-releasing factor; LH = luteinizing hormone; P = progesterone.

V Male Gametogenesis (Spermatogenesis) (Figure 1-3) is classically divided into three phases: spermatocytogenesis, meiosis, and spermiogenesis.

A. SPERMATOCYTOGENESIS

1. **Primordial germ cells (46,2N)** from the wall of the yolk sac arrive in the testes at week 6 of embryonic development and remain dormant until puberty.
2. At puberty, primordial germ cells differentiate into **type A spermatogonia** (46,2N).
3. Type A spermatogonia undergo **mitosis** to provide a continuous supply of stem cells throughout the reproductive life of the male (called spermatocytogenesis).
4. Some type A spermatogonia differentiate into **type B spermatogonia** (46,2N).

B. MEIOSIS

1. Type B spermatogonia enter meiosis I and undergo DNA replication to form **primary spermatocytes** (46,4N).
2. Primary spermatocytes complete meiosis I to form two **secondary spermatocytes** (23,2N).
3. Secondary spermatocytes complete meiosis II to form four **spermatids** (23,1N).

C. SPERMIOGENESIS

1. Spermatids undergo a **postmeiotic series of morphological changes** (called spermiogenesis) to form **sperm** (23,1N).
2. Newly ejaculated sperm are incapable of fertilization until they undergo **capacitation**, which occurs in the female reproductive tract and involves the unmasking of sperm glycosyltransferases and removal of proteins coating the surface of the sperm.

VI Clinical Considerations

A. OFFSPRING OF OLDER WOMEN

1. Prolonged dormancy of primary oocytes may be the reason for the high incidence of chromosomal abnormalities in offspring of older women. Since all primary oocytes are formed by month 5 of fetal life, a female infant is born with her entire supply of gametes. Primary oocytes remain dormant until ovulation; those ovulated late in the woman's reproductive life may have been dormant for as long as 40 years.
2. The incidence of **trisomy 21 (Down syndrome)** increases with advanced age of the mother. The primary cause of Down syndrome is maternal meiotic nondisjunction. Clinical findings include severe mental retardation, epicanthal folds, Brushfield spots, simian creases, and association with a decrease in α-fetoprotein.

B. OFFSPRING OF OLDER MEN.

An increased incidence of **achondroplasia** (an autosomal dominant congenital skeletal anomaly characterized by retarded bone growth in the limbs with normal-sized head and trunk) and **Marfan syndrome** are associated with advanced paternal age.

C. MALE INFERTILITY

1. **Sperm number and motility:** Infertile males produce less than 10 million sperm/mL of semen. Fertile males produce from 20 to more than 100 million sperm/mL of semen. Normally up to 10% of sperm in an ejaculate may be grossly deformed (two heads or two tails), but these sperm probably do not fertilize an oocyte owing to their lack of motility.

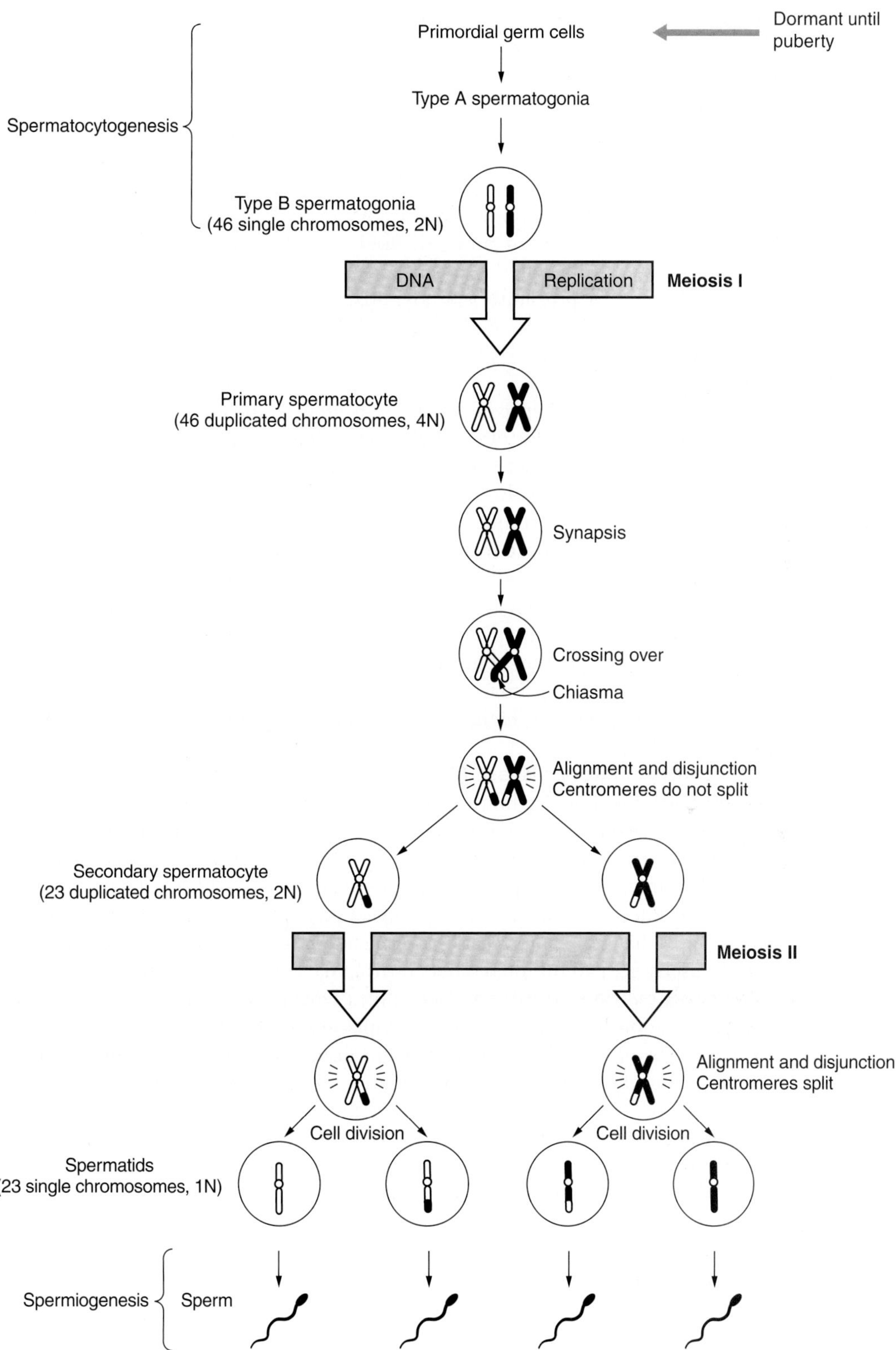

● **Figure 1-3 Male gametogenesis (spermatogenesis).** Note that only one pair of homologous chromosomes is shown (white = maternal origin; black = paternal origin). Synapsis is the process of pairing of homologous chromosomes. The point at which the DNA molecule crosses over is called the chiasma and is where exchange of small amounts of maternal and paternal DNA occurs. Note that synapsis and crossing over occur only during meiosis I.

2. **Hypogonadotropic hypogonadism** is a condition where the hypothalamus produces reduced levels of GnRF leading to reduced levels of FSH and LH and finally reduced levels of testosterone. **Kallmann syndrome** is a genetic disorder characterized by hypogonadotropic hypogonadism and anosmia (loss of smell).
3. **Drugs:** Cancer chemotherapy, anabolic steroids, cimetidine (histamine H_2-receptor antagonist that inhibits stomach HCl production), spironolactone (a K^+-sparing diuretic), phenytoin (an antiepileptic drug), sulfasalazine (a sulfa drug used to treat ulcerative colitis, Crohn's disease, rheumatoid arthritis, and psoriatic arthritis), and nitrofurantoin (an antibiotic used to treat urinary tract infections).
4. **Other factors:** Klinefelter syndrome, seminoma, cryptochordism, varicocele, hydrocele, mumps, prostatitis, epididymitis, hypospadias, ductus deferens obstruction, and impotence.

D. FEMALE INFERTILITY

1. **Anovulation** is the absence of ovulation in some women due to inadequate secretion of FSH and LH and is often treated with **clomiphene citrate** (a fertility drug). Clomiphene citrate competes with estrogen for binding sites in the adenohypophysis, thereby suppressing the normal negative feedback loop of estrogen on the adenohypophysis. This stimulates FSH and LH secretion and induces ovulation.
2. **Premature ovarian failure (primary ovarian insufficiency)** is the loss of function of the ovaries before age 40, resulting in infertility. The cause is generally idiopathic, but cases have been attributed to autoimmune disorders, Turner syndrome, Fragile X syndrome, chemotherapy, or radiation treatment. The age of onset can be seen in early teenage years, but varies widely. If a girl never begins menstruation, the condition is called **primary ovarian failure**. Clinical findings include: amenorrhea, low estrogen levels, high FSH levels, and ultrasound may show small ovaries without follicles.
3. **Pelvic inflammatory disease (PID)** refers to the infection of the uterus, uterine tubes, and/or ovaries leading to inflammation and scar formation. The cause is generally a sexually transmitted infection (STI), usually Neisseria gonorrhea or Chlamydia trachomatis. However, many other routes are possible (lymphatic spread, hematogenous spread, postpartum infections, postabortal [miscarriage or abortion] infections, or intrauterine device infections). Clinical findings include: some cases that are asymptomatic, fever, tenderness of the cervix, lower abdominal pain, discharge, painful intercourse, or irregular menstrual bleeding.
4. **Polycystic ovarian syndrome** is a complex female endocrine disorder defined by oligo-ovulation (infrequent, irregular ovulations), androgen excess, multiple ovarian cysts (by ultrasound). The cause is uncertain, but a strong genetic component exists. Clinical findings include: anovulation, irregular menstruation, amenorrhea, ovulation-related infertility, high androgen levels or activity resulting in acne and hirsutism, insulin resistance associated with obesity, and Type II diabetes.
5. **Endometriosis** is the appearance of foci of endometrial tissue in abnormal locations outside the uterus (e.g., ovary, uterine ligaments, pelvic peritoneum). The ectopic endometrial tissue shows cyclic hormonal changes synchronous with the cyclic hormonal changes of the endometrium in the uterus. Clinical findings include: infertility, dysmenorrhea, pelvic pain (most pronounced at the time of menstruation), dysuria, painful sex, and throbbing pain in the legs.

Chapter **2**

Week 1 (Days 1–7)*

I Overview.

Figure 2-1 summarizes the events that occur during week 1, following fertilization.

II Fertilization

A. Occurs in the **ampulla of the uterine tube**.

B. The sperm binds to the zona pellucida of the secondary oocyte arrested in metaphase of meiosis II and triggers the **acrosome reaction**, causing the release of acrosomal enzymes (e.g., **acrosin**).

C. Aided by the acrosomal enzymes, the sperm penetrates the zona pellucida. Penetration of the zona pellucida elicits the **cortical reaction**. The cortical reaction is the release of lysosomal enzymes from cortical granules near the oocyte cell membrane that changes the oocyte cell membrane potential and inactivates sperm receptors on the zona pellucida.

D. These changes are called the **polyspermy block**, which is thought to render the secondary oocyte impermeable to other sperm. However, we know that polyspermy block does not work very well since diandric triploidy (an embryo with three sets of chromosomes, two of which come from the father) is quite common.

E. The sperm and secondary oocyte cell membranes fuse. The nuclear contents and the centriole pair of the sperm enter the cytoplasm of the oocyte. The sperm nuclear contents form the **male pronucleus**. The tail and mitochondria of the sperm degenerate. Therefore, all mitochondria within the zygote are of maternal origin (i.e., **all mitochondrial DNA is of maternal origin**). The oocyte loses its centriole pair during meiosis so that the establishment of a functional zygote depends on the sperm centriole pair (a cardinal feature of human embryogenesis) to produce a microtubule organizing center (MTOC).

F. The secondary oocyte completes meiosis II, forming a mature **ovum**. The nucleus of the ovum is the **female pronucleus**.

*The age of the developing conceptus can be measured either from the estimated day of fertilization (fertilization age) or from the day of the last normal menstrual period (LNMP). In this book, ages are presented as fertilization age.

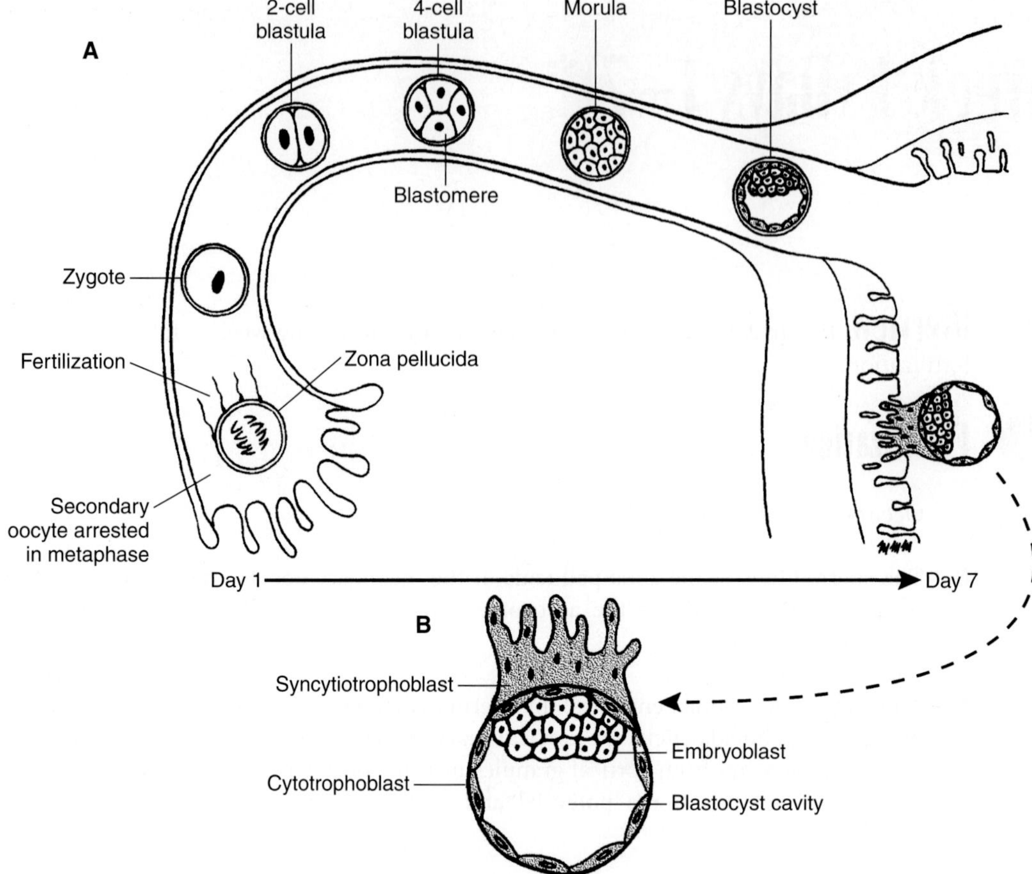

● **Figure 2-1 (A)** The stages of human development during week 1. **(B)** A day 7 blastocyst.

G. **Syngamy** is a term that describes the successful completion of fertilization, that is, the formation of a **zygote.** Syngamy occurs when the male and female pronuclei fuse and the cytoplasmic machinery for proper cell division exists.

H. The life span of a zygote is only a few hours because its existence terminates when the first cleavage division occurs.

III Cleavage

A. Cleavage is a series of **mitotic** divisions of the zygote, where the plane of the first mitotic division passes through the area of the cell membrane where the polar bodies were previously extruded.

B. In humans, cleavage is **holoblastic**, which means the cells divide completely through their cytoplasm. Cleavage is **asymmetrical**, which means the daughter cells are unequal in size (i.e., one cell gets more cytoplasm than the other) at least during the first few cell divisions. Cleavage is **asynchronous**, which means only one cell will divide at a time;

generally the largest daughter cell will divide next at least during the first few cell divisions.

C. The process of cleavage eventually forms a **blastula**, consisting of cells called **blastomeres**.

D. A cluster of blastomeres (16–32 blastomeres) forms a **morula**.

E. Blastomeres are **totipotent** up to the eight-cell stage (i.e., each blastomere can form a complete embryo by itself). **Totipotency** refers to a stem cell that can differentiate into every cell within the organism, including extraembryonic tissues.

IV Blastocyst Formation

A. Occurs when fluid secreted within the morula forms the **blastocyst cavity**.

B. The inner cell mass, which becomes the **embryo**, is called the **embryoblast**. The embryoblast cells are **pluripotent**. **Pluripotency** refers to a stem cell that can differentiate into ectoderm, mesoderm, and endoderm.

C. The outer cell mass, which becomes part of the **placenta**, is called the **trophoblast**.

V Implantation

A. The **zona pellucida must degenerate** for implantation to occur.

B. The blastocyst implants within the **posterior superior wall** of the uterus.

C. The blastocyst implants within the **functional layer of the endometrium** during the **secretory phase** of the menstrual cycle.

D. The trophoblast differentiates into **cytotrophoblast** and **syncytiotrophoblast**.

VI Clinical Considerations

A. ECTOPIC TUBAL PREGNANCY (ETP)

1. An ETP occurs when the blastocyst implants within the uterine tube due to **delayed transport**. The **ampulla of uterine tube** is the most common site of an ETP. The **rectouterine pouch (pouch of Douglas)** is a common site for an ectopic abdominal pregnancy.
2. An ETP is frequently predisposed by **chronic salpingitis**, **endometriosis**, and **postoperative adhesions**.
3. An ETP is most commonly seen in women with **endometriosis** or **pelvic inflammatory disease**.
4. An ETP leads to uterine tube rupture and hemorrhage if surgical intervention (i.e., salpingectomy) is not performed.

5. An ETP must be differentially diagnosed from **appendicitis**, an **aborting intrauterine pregnancy**, or a **bleeding corpus luteum** of a normal intrauterine pregnancy.
6. Clinical signs of an ETP include: **abnormal uterine bleeding, unilateral pelvic pain, increased levels of human chorionic gonadotropin (hCG)** (but lower than originally expected with uterine implantation pregnancy), and a **massive first-trimester bleed**.

B. TWINNING (FIGURE 2-2)

1. Steps in monozygotic (identical) twinning

a. A secondary oocyte arrested in metaphase of meiosis II is fertilized by one sperm. The nuclear contents and centriole pair of the sperm enter the oocyte cytoplasm.
b. The secondary oocyte completes meiosis II, forming the second polar body. The female and male pronuclei form.
c. The female and male pronuclei fuse and the centriole pair provides the cytoplasmic machinery for cleavage cell divisions to occur. A zygote is formed.
d. Cleavage divisions produce a cluster of blastomeres called a morula surrounded by a zona pellucida. The molecular mechanisms that establish twin embryogenesis are active in the morula and are responsible for the latter "splitting" of the inner cell mass. In other words, twinning causes the "splitting," not vice versa. The twinning morula can travel two different routes leading to either monochorionic or dichorionic twins.
e. If "splitting" occurs AFTER the differentiation of the trophoblast, then monochorionic twins will form.
f. If "splitting" occurs BEFORE the differentiation of the trophoblast, then dichorionic twins will form.

2. Steps in dizygotic (fraternal) twinning

a. A secondary oocyte arrested in metaphase of meiosis II is fertilized by two sperm. The nuclear contents and centriole pair of both sperm enter the oocyte cytoplasm.
b. The secondary oocyte completes meiosis II, but does not form a secondary polar body. Instead, the DNA that would have been sequestered in second polar body forms another female pronucleus. There are now two separate cellular entities within the zona pellucida each containing a female and male pronucleus.
c. The female and male pronuclei fuse and the centriole pair provides the cytoplasmic machinery for cleavage cell divisions to occur. Two zygotes are formed with two different genotypes.
d. Cleavage divisions produce a cluster of blastomeres called a morula surrounded by a zona pellucida. The morula is a **chimera** consisting of an assortment of cells with two different genotypes. The molecular mechanisms that establish twin embryogenesis are active in the chimeric morula and are responsible for the latter "splitting" of the inner cell mass. In other words, twinning causes the "splitting," not vice versa. The twinning chimeric morula can travel two different routes leading to either monochorionic or dichorionic twins.
e. If "splitting" occurs AFTER the differentiation of the trophoblast, then monochorionic twins will form.
f. If "splitting" occurs BEFORE the differentiation of the trophoblast, then dichorionic twins will form.

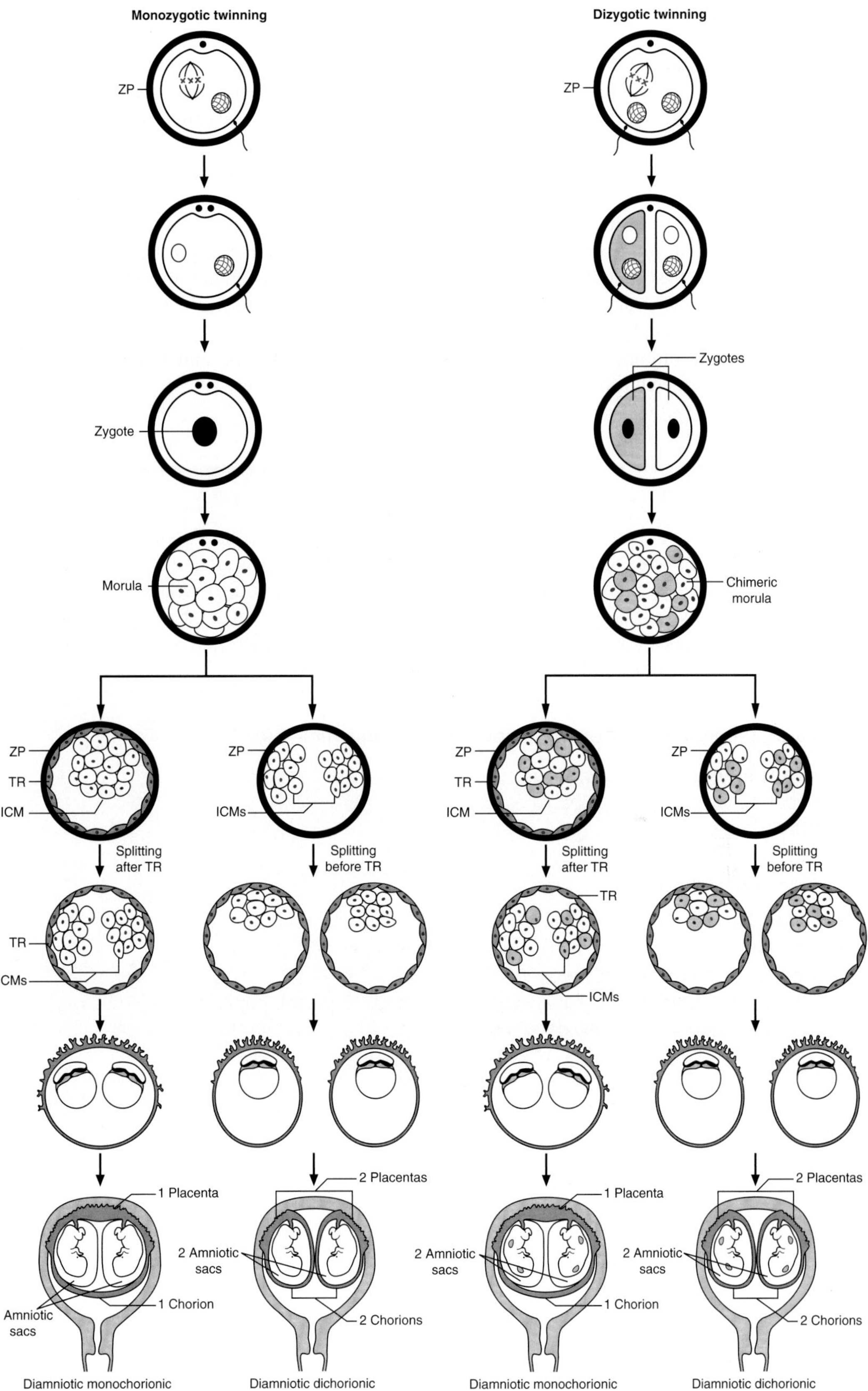

● **Figure 2-2** Diagram of monozygotic and dizygotic twinning. ZP = zona pellucida; TR = trophoblast; ICM = inner cell mass.

3. Conjoined (Siamese) twinning

a. Occurs exactly like monozygotic twins except that there is incomplete "splitting" of the inner cell mass. The exact molecular mechanisms involved are not clear.

b. All conjoined twins (except parasitic twins) are symmetrical (i.e., like parts are fused to like parts).

c. The most common types of conjoined twins are: (1) thoraco-omphalopagus (fusion from upper chest to lower chest), (2) thoracopagus (fusion from upper chest to lower abdomen), (3) omphalopagus (fusion at lower chest), craniopagus (fusion of skulls), and parasitic twins (asymmetrically conjoined; one twin is small and dependent on the larger twin).

d. Conjoined twins are monoamniotic (i.e., one amnion) and monochorionic (i.e., one chorion).

Case Study 1

A 25-year-old woman comes into your office complaining of "spotting" and having "stomach pains" as she points to her lower abdominal area. She noted that she and her husband were trying to have a baby and that she had her last period about 5 weeks ago. She said that after talking with her girlfriends about her symptoms, she was a little afraid of what it could be, so she decided to see a physician. Her chart shows that she has had a history of pelvic inflammatory disease. What is the most likely diagnosis?

Differentials

- Ectopic pregnancy, spontaneous abortion, pelvic inflammatory disease

Relevant Physical Exam Findings

- Tender pelvic mass was palpable
- Amenorrhea
- Light vaginal bleeding
- Lower abdominal pain

Relevant Lab Findings

- Elevated β-hCG but lower than expected for pregnancy
- Lower-than-normal progesterone
- Absence of intrauterine pregnancy on ultrasound. However, implantation in the ampulla of the left uterine tube was detected.

Diagnosis

- Ectopic pregnancy

Case Study 2

A 32-year-old woman comes into the emergency room in the evening complaining of shortness of breath. The episode began suddenly earlier in the day. She also tells you that for the last few days she has had abdominal pain but cannot point to a specific area. She says that "my stomach feels distended, I'm nauseous, and I've been vomiting for the last few days." And "it's worse at night when I lie down and when I take a deep breath." After talking to her for awhile, you learn that she and her husband have been trying to start a family for long time with no success. So she recently started the procedure for in vitro fertilization. She underwent controlled ovarian stimulation with gonadotropins achieving a peak estradiol level of 4500 pg/mL three weeks ago followed by embryo transfer 1 week ago prior to coming into the emergency room.

Differentials

- Atrial fibrillation, pulmonary embolism, coronary artery disease, gastric ulcer, ectopic pregnancy

Relevant Physical Exam Findings

- Awake, alert, but in moderate distress
- Heart rate: 108 bpm
- Heart is regular, tachycardiac, and without murmurs
- Respiratory rate: 26 breaths/minute (rapid, shallow breathing)
- Bilaterally decreased breath sounds
- Abdomen is distended with normal bowel sounds
- Moderate tenderness throughout the abdomen with ascites

Relevant Lab Findings

- Hemoglobin: 16.8 g/dL (high); Hematocrit: 49.7% (high); WBC: 12.9 × 10^9/L (high); Na^+: 130 mEq/L (low); K^+: 5.6 mEq/L (high)
- Chest radiograph shows bilateral pleural effusions
- Ultrasonograph shows a large ovarian volume with ascites

Diagnosis

- Ovarian Hyperstimulation Syndrome (OHSS): OHSS is a known complication of in vitro fertilization with a prevalence of 3.4% for moderate OHSS and 1% for severe OHSS. OHSS is caused by high levels of vascular endothelial growth factor (VEGF) produced by the enlarged and luteinized ovaries. VEGF is a vasoactive substance that causes leaky capillaries, which shifts fluid out of the intravascular space causing pleural effusions, pulmonary edema, or ascites. OHSS is a self-limiting complication and usually resolves within 1 week. The treatment of OHSS is primarily supportive and includes gradual rehydration with saline, electrolyte normalization, and discontinuation of fertility agents. There is an increased risk for a thromboembolism, so heparin treatment may be indicated. Since 1 out of 6 couples face infertility issues and the demand for in vitro fertilization is on the rise due to delayed childbearing by the woman, physicians need to become aware of this complication.

Chapter **3**

Week 2 (Days 8–14)

I Embryoblast (Figure 3-1)

A. The embryoblast differentiates into two distinct cell layers: the dorsal **epiblast** and the ventral **hypoblast**. The epiblast and hypoblast together form a flat, ovoid-shaped disk known as the **bilaminar embryonic disk**.

B. Within the epiblast, clefts develop and eventually coalesce to form the **amniotic cavity**.

C. Hypoblast cells migrate and line the inner surface of the cytotrophoblast and eventually delimit a space called the definitive **yolk sac**.

D. The epiblast and hypoblast fuse to form the **prochordal plate**, which marks the future site of the **mouth**.

II Trophoblast

A. The syncytiotrophoblast continues its growth into the endometrium to make contact with endometrial blood vessels and glands.

B. The syncytiotrophoblast **does not divide mitotically**. The cytotrophoblast does divide mitotically, adding to the growth of the syncytiotrophoblast.

C. The syncytiotrophoblast produces **human chorionic gonadotropin (hCG)**.

D. **Primary chorionic villi** formed by the cytotrophoblast protrude into the syncytiotrophoblast.

III Extraembryonic Mesoderm

A. Is a new layer of cells derived from the epiblast.

B. **Extraembryonic somatic mesoderm (somatopleuric mesoderm)** lines the cytotrophoblast, forms the **connecting stalk**, and covers the amnion (see Figure 3-1).

C. The conceptus is suspended by the connecting stalk within the **chorionic cavity**.

D. The wall of the chorionic cavity is called the **chorion** and consists of three components: **extraembryonic somatic mesoderm**, **cytotrophoblast**, and **syncytiotrophoblast**.

E. **Extraembryonic visceral mesoderm (splanchnopleuric mesoderm)** covers the yolk sac.

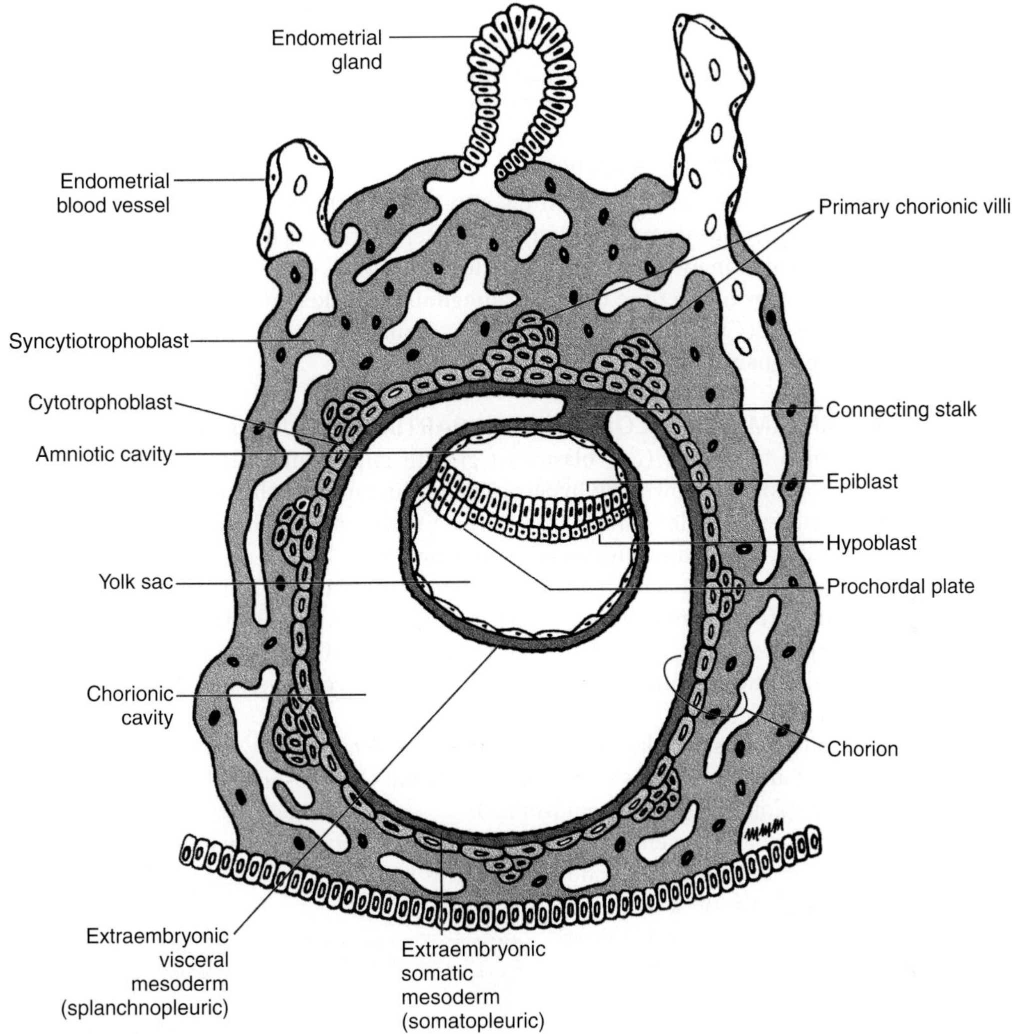

● **Figure 3-1** A day 14 blastocyst, highlighting the formation of the bilaminar embryonic disk and the completion of implantation within the endometrium.

IV Clinical Considerations

A. HUMAN CHORIONIC GONADOTROPIN

1. hCG is a glycoprotein produced by the syncytiotrophoblast that stimulates the production of progesterone by the corpus luteum of the ovary (i.e., maintains corpus luteum function). This is clinically significant because progesterone produced by the corpus luteum is essential for the maintenance of pregnancy until week 8. The placenta then takes over progesterone production.
2. hCG can be assayed in **maternal blood at day 8** or **maternal urine at day 10** and is the basis of pregnancy testing.
3. hCG is detectable throughout a pregnancy.

4. **Low hCG values** may predict a spontaneous abortion or indicate an ectopic pregnancy.
5. **High hCG values** may indicate a multiple pregnancy, hydatidiform mole, or gestational trophoblastic neoplasia (GTN) (such as choriocarcinoma).

B. RU-486 (MIFEPRISTONE; MIFEPREX)

1. Will initiate menstruation when taken within 8–10 weeks of the start of the last menstrual period. If implantation of a conceptus has occurred, the conceptus will be sloughed along with the endometrium.
2. RU-486 is a **progesterone-receptor antagonist (blocker)** used in conjunction with **misoprostol (Cytotec; a prostaglandin E_1 analogue)** and is 96% effective at terminating pregnancy.

C. HYDATIDIFORM MOLE (COMPLETE OR PARTIAL) (FIGURE 3-2)

1. A blighted blastocyst (i.e., blastocyst growth is prevented) leads to death of the embryo. This is followed by hyperplastic proliferation of the trophoblast.
2. A hydatidiform mole (complete or partial) represents an abnormal placenta characterized by marked enlargement of chorionic villi.
3. A complete mole usually has an apparently normal 46,XX karyotype, but both nuclear chromosomes are of paternal origin. This results from fertilization of an "empty" egg (i.e., absent or inactivated maternal chromosomes) by a haploid sperm that then duplicates (46,YY moles do not occur, because this karyotype is lethal).
4. A partial mole usually has a triploid karyotype (69,XXX; 69,XXY) due to the fertilization of an ovum (one set of haploid maternal chromosomes) by two sperm (two sets of haploid paternal chromosomes).
5. A complete mole (no embryo present) is distinguished from a partial mole (embryo present) by the amount of chorionic villous involvement.
6. The hallmarks of a complete mole include gross, generalized edema of chorionic villi forming grape-like, transparent vesicles, hyperplastic proliferation of surrounding trophoblastic cells, and absence of an embryo/fetus.
7. Clinical signs diagnostic of a mole include preeclampsia during the first trimester, elevated hCG levels (>100,000 mIU/mL), and an enlarged uterus with bleeding.
8. Follow-up visits after a mole are essential because 3%–5% of moles develop into GTN.
9. Figure 3-2 shows a hydatidiform mole with gross edema of the chorionic villi forming grape-like vesicles.

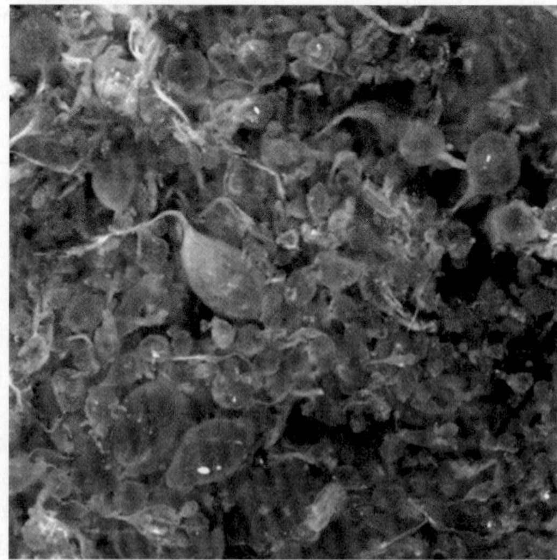

● **Figure 3-2** A hydatidiform mole.

D. GESTATIONAL TROPHOBLASTIC NEOPLASIA OR CHORIOCARCINOMA (FIGURE 3-3)

1. GTN is a malignant tumor of the trophoblast that may occur following a normal or ectopic pregnancy, abortion, or a hydatidiform mole.
2. With a high degree of suspicion, elevated hCG levels are diagnostic.
3. Nonmetastatic GTN (i.e., confined to the uterus) is the most common form of the neoplasia, and treatment is highly successful. However, the prognosis of metastatic GTN is poor if it spreads to the liver or brain.
4. Figure 3-3 shows hemorrhagic nodules metastatic to the liver. This is due to the rapid proliferation of trophoblastic cells combined with marked propensity to invade blood vessels. The central portion of the lesion is hemorrhagic and necrotic with only a thin rim of trophoblastic cells at the periphery.

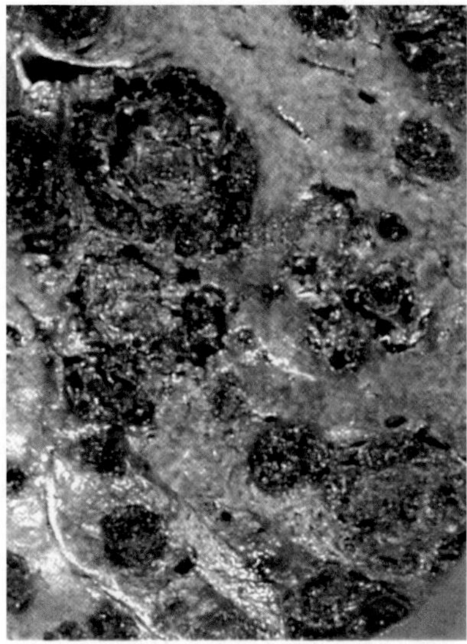

● **Figure 3-3** Hemorrhagic nodules metastatic to the liver.

Case Study

A 31-year-old woman comes into the office complaining of "running a fever," being nauseated, and losing weight, "about 15 lb or so," over the last month. She tells you that she had a miscarriage about 2 months ago and "all of a sudden these other problems come up." She adds that the doctors said she had "preeclampsia" during her first trimester of that pregnancy. She said that she was supposed to come back in but she didn't because she "felt depressed about losing the baby." She remarks that she hasn't had any changes in her diet and that she "thought she would have gained weight with all the food she was eating." What is the most likely diagnosis?

Differentials

- Malnutrition, loss of appetite, achalasia, hyperthyroidism, cachexia from a malignant tumor

Relevant Physical Exam Findings

- Normal thyroid on palpation
- No coughing blood
- No diarrhea

Relevant Lab Findings

- Elevated hCG

Diagnosis

- Choriocarcinoma: This is a result from her premalignant condition of hydatidiform mole, which presents with preeclampsia during the first trimester and elevated hCG, progressing to a GTN. Malnutrition and loss of appetite were excluded because she mentioned that she was eating a lot of food. Hyperthyroidism was excluded because there was no mention of elevated thyroid-stimulating hormone (TSH).

Chapter **4**

Embryonic Period (Weeks 3–8)

I Introduction.

Introduction. All major organ systems begin to develop during the embryonic period, causing a **craniocaudal** and **lateral body folding** of the embryo. By the end of the embryonic period (week 8), the embryo has a distinct human appearance. During the embryonic period, the basic segmentation of the human embryo in a craniocaudal direction is controlled by the **Hox (homeobox) complex** of genes. Embryogenesis proceeds at a slower pace in female embryos due to the presence of the paternally imprinted X chromosome.

II Gastrulation (Figure 4-1)

A. Is a process that establishes the three primary germ layers (**ectoderm**, **mesoderm**, and **endoderm**), thereby forming a **trilaminar embryonic disk**.

B. This process is first indicated by the formation of the **primitive streak** in the midline of the epiblast. As early as the bilaminar and trilaminar stages of embryogenesis, left side/right side (L/R) axis determination begins with the asymmetric activity **sonic hedgehog protein (Shh)** only on the future left side since Shh activity is suppressed on the future right side by **activin**. In addition, the neurotransmitter **serotonin (5HT)** plays an important role in L/R axis determination. After L/R axis determination, the L/R asymmetry of a number of organs (e.g., heart, liver, stomach) can be patterned by the embryo.

C. Ectoderm gives further rise to **neuroectoderm** and **neural crest cells**.

D. Endoderm remains intact.

E. Mesoderm gives further rise to **paraxial mesoderm** (somitomeres and 35 pairs of somites), **intermediate mesoderm**, and **lateral mesoderm.**

F. The somites segment into the **sclerotome** (forms axial **cartilage and bone**), **myotome** (forms axial **muscle**), and the **dermatome** (forms the **dermis of skin**).

G. The intermediate mesoderm forms the **urogenital system**.

H. The lateral mesoderm is split into two layers by the formation of the intraembryonic coelom called the **somatic layer** and the **splanchnic layer**. The somatic layer of the lateral mesoderm and the ectoderm form the embryonic body wall or **somatopleure**. The visceral layer of the lateral mesoderm and the endoderm form the embryonic gut tube or **splanchnopleure**.

I. All adult cells and tissues can trace their embryological origin back to the three primary germ layers (see Table 4-1).

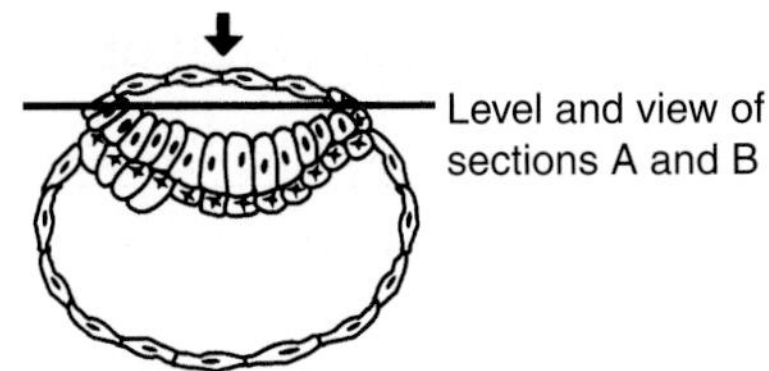

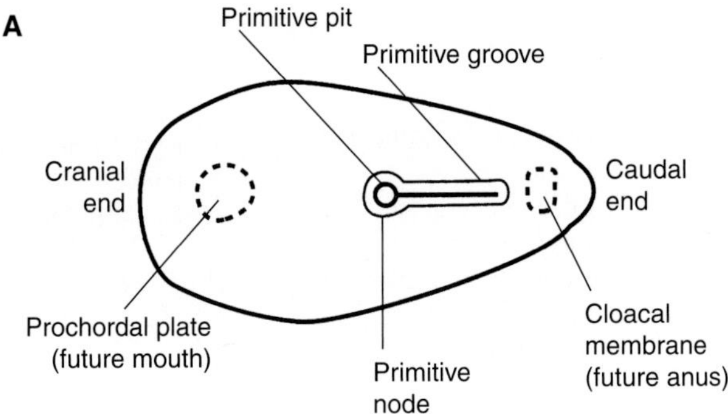

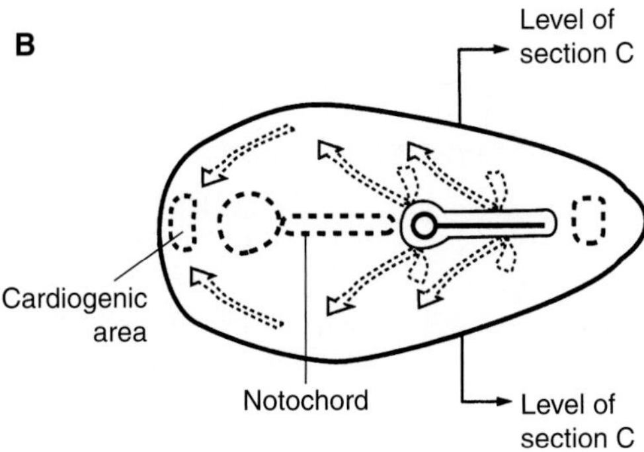

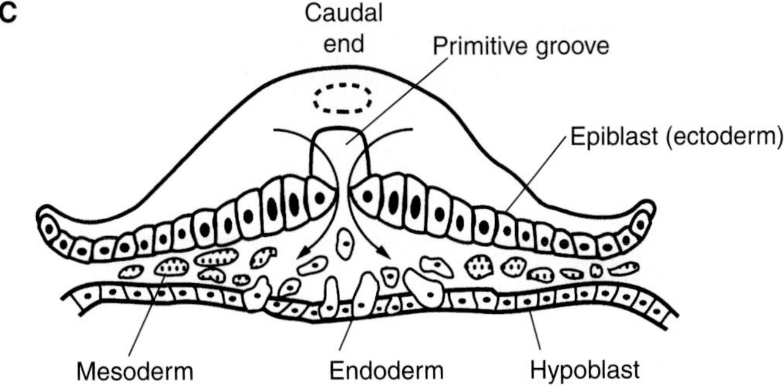

● **Figure 4-1 Gastrulation.** The embryoblast in the upper left is provided for orientation. **(A)** Dorsal view of the epiblast. The primitive streak consists of the primitive groove, node, and pit. **(B)** Arrows show the migration of cells through the primitive streak. The notochord (i.e., mesoderm located between the primitive node and prochordal plate) induces the formation of the neural tube. The cardiogenic area is the future site of the heart. **(C)** Epiblast cells migrate to the primitive streak and insert themselves between the epiblast and the hypoblast. Some epiblast cells displace the hypoblast to form endoderm; the remainder migrates cranially, laterally, and along the midline to form mesoderm. After gastrulation, the epiblast is called ectoderm.

TABLE 4-1 PARTIAL LIST OF GERM LAYER DERIVATIVES

Ectoderm	Mesoderm	Endoderm
Epidermis, hair, nails, sweat and sebaceous glands Adenohypophysis **Epithelial lining of the:** Lower anal canal Distal part of male urethra External auditory meatus	Muscle (smooth, cardiac, and skeletal) Muscles of tongue (occipital somites) Pharyngeal arch muscles (muscles of mastication, muscles of facial expression) Connective tissue Dermis and subcutaneous layer of skin Bone and cartilage Dura mater Endothelium of blood vessels RBCs, WBCs, microglia, and Kupffer cells Kidney Adrenal cortex	Hepatocytes Acinar and islet cells of pancreas **Epithelial lining of the:** GI tract Trachea, bronchi, lungs Biliary apparatus Urinary bladder Female urethra Most of male urethra Inferior two-thirds of vagina Auditory tube, middle ear cavity
Neuroectoderm All neurons within brain and spinal cord (CNS) Retina Optic nerve (CN II) Dilator and sphincter pupillae muscles Astrocytes, oligodendrocytes, ependymocytes, tanycytes, choroid plexus cells Neurohypophysis Pineal gland		
Neural crest Neurons within ganglia (dorsal root, cranial, autonomic) Schwann cells Pia and arachnoid Adrenal medulla Melanocytes Aorticopulmonary septum Bones of the neurocranium Pharyngeal arch bones (maxilla, mandible, malleus, incus)		

CN = cranial nerve; CNS = central nervous system; GI = gastrointestinal; RBCs = red blood cells; WBCs = white blood cells.

III Clinical Considerations

A. CHORDOMA (CD)

1. Is either a benign or malignant tumor that arises from remnants of the **notochord**.
2. CD may be found either intracranially or in the sacral region and occurs more commonly in men late in adult life (age 50 years).

B. FIRST MISSED MENSTRUAL PERIOD

1. Is usually the **first indication of pregnancy**.
2. Week 3 of embryonic development coincides with the first missed menstrual period. Note that at this time the embryo has already undergone 2 weeks of development.
3. It is crucial that the woman become aware of a pregnancy as soon as possible because the embryonic period is a period of **high susceptibility to teratogens**.

C. SELECTIVE SEROTONIN REUPTAKE INHIBITORS (SSRIS)

1. Children whose mothers have been treated for depression with SSRIs have an increased risk of heart malformations.
2. This is probably due to the role of serotonin in L/R axis determination.

D. SACROCOCCYGEAL TERATOMA (ST; FIGURE 4-2)

1. Is a tumor that arises from remnants of the **primitive streak**, which normally degenerates and disappears.
2. ST is derived from pluripotent cells of the primitive streak and often contains various types of tissue (e.g., bone, nerve, hair).
3. ST occurs more commonly in female infants and usually becomes malignant during infancy (must be removed by age 6 months). Figure 4-2 shows an infant with a sacrococcygeal teratoma.

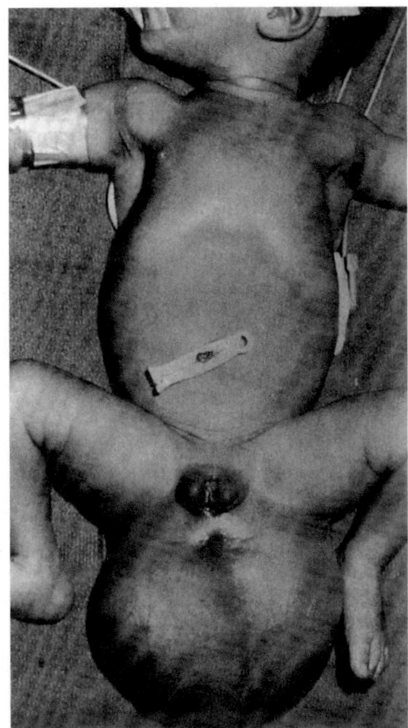

● **Figure 4-2** Sacrococcygeal teratoma.

E. CAUDAL DYSPLASIA (SIRENOMELIA; FIGURE 4-3)

1. Refers to a constellation of syndromes ranging from minor lesions of lower vertebrae to complete fusion of the lower limbs.
2. Caudal dysplasia is caused by abnormal gastrulation, in which the migration of mesoderm is disturbed. It can be associated with various cranial anomalies.
3. **VATER,** which includes vertebral defects, anal atresia, tracheoesophageal fistula, and renal defects.
4. **VACTERL,** which is similar to VATER but also includes cardiovascular defects and upper limb defects. Figure 4-3 shows an infant with caudal dysplasia (sirenomelia).

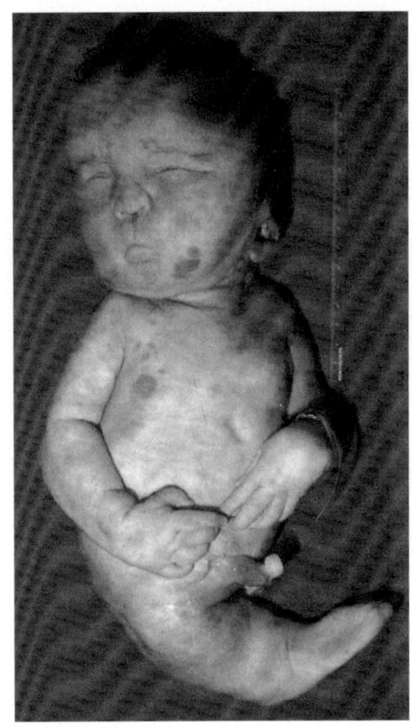

● **Figure 4-3** Caudal dysplasia (sirenomelia).

Case Study

A distraught mother brings her 2-month-old daughter into your office saying that she noticed a "lump growing from her child's bottom." She states she "noticed it about 2 weeks ago while changing her daughter's diaper"; it was small and so she didn't think much of it, and over time, it has "grown to the size of a baseball." What is the most likely diagnosis?

Differentials

- Sacrococcygeal teratoma, spina bifida with meningocele, spina bifida with meningomyelocele

Relevant Physical Exam Findings

- Large spheroid size mass that appears to be very firm upon palpation

Relevant Lab Findings

- Biopsy of the mass shows tissue containing hair, teeth, muscle fibers, and thyroid follicular cells

Diagnosis

- Sacrococcygeal teratoma is a remnant of the primitive streak that contains all three germ layers: ectoderm (hair and teeth), mesoderm (muscle fibers), and endoderm (thyroid follicular cells). A sacrococcygeal teratoma is different from spina bifida with meningocele or spina bifida with meningomyelocele, which is a failure of the bony vertebral arches to fuse with the protrusion of cerebrospinal fluid–filled sac.

Chapter 5

Placenta, Amniotic Fluid, and Umbilical Cord

I Placenta (Figure 5-1)

- The placenta is formed when the embryo invades the endometrium of the uterus and when the trophoblast forms the villous chorion.
- Villous chorion formation goes through three stages: **primary chorionic villi**, **secondary chorionic villi**, and **tertiary chorionic villi**.

A. COMPONENTS

1. The maternal component of the placenta

a. Consists of the **decidua basalis**, which is derived from the endometrium of the uterus located between the blastocyst and the myometrium.

b. The decidua basalis and **decidua parietalis** (which includes all portions of the endometrium other than the site of implantation) are shed as part of the afterbirth.

c. The **decidua capsularis**, the portion of endometrium that covers the blastocyst and separates it from the uterine cavity, becomes attenuated and degenerates at week 22 of development because of a reduced blood supply.

d. The **maternal surface** of the placenta is characterized by 8–10 compartments called **cotyledons** (imparting a **cobblestone appearance**), which are separated by decidual (placental) septa.

e. The maternal surface is **dark red in color and oozes blood** due to torn maternal blood vessels.

2. The fetal component of the placenta

a. Consists of **tertiary chorionic villi** derived from both the trophoblast and extraembryonic mesoderm, which collectively become known as the **villous chorion.**

b. The villous chorion develops most prolifically at the site of the decidua basalis. The villous chorion is in contrast to an area of no villus development known as the **smooth chorion** (which is related to the decidua capsularis).

c. The **fetal surface** of the placenta is characterized by the well-vascularized chorionic plate containing the chorionic (fetal) blood vessels.

d. The fetal surface has a **smooth, shiny, light-blue or blue-pink appearance** (because the amnion covers the fetal surface), and 5–8 **large chorionic (fetal) blood vessels** should be apparent.

B. CLINICAL CONSIDERATIONS

1. Velamentous placenta occurs when the **umbilical (fetal) blood vessels** abnormally travel through the amniochorionic membrane before reaching the placenta proper. If the umbilical (fetal) blood vessels cross the internal os, a serious condition called **vasa previa** exists. In vasa previa, if one of the umbilical (fetal) blood vessels ruptures during pregnancy, labor, or delivery, the fetus will bleed to death.

2. **Placenta previa** occurs when the placenta attaches in the lower part of the uterus, **covering the internal os.** The placenta normally implants in the posterior superior wall of the uterus. **Uterine (maternal) blood vessels** rupture during the later part of pregnancy as the uterus begins to gradually dilate. The mother may bleed to death, and the fetus will also be placed in jeopardy because of the compromised blood supply. Because the placenta blocks the cervical opening, delivery is usually accomplished by cesarean section (C-section). This condition is clinically associated with **repeated episodes of bright-red vaginal bleeding**. Placenta previa is the classic cause of **third-trimester bleeding**, whereas an ectopic pregnancy is the classic cause of first-trimester bleeding.
3. **Placenta accreta/increta/percreta** occurs when a placenta implants on the myometrium, deep into the myometrium, or through the wall of the uterus, respectively. This results in retained placenta and hemorrhage and may lead to uterine rupture (placenta percreta). Risk factors include multiple curettages, previous C-sections, severe endometritis, or closely spaced pregnancies.
4. **Preeclampsia and eclampsia.** Severe preeclampsia refers to the sudden development of **maternal hypertension (>160/110 mm Hg)**, **edema (hands and/or face)**, and **proteinuria (>5 g/24 hr)** usually after week 32 of gestation (third trimester). Eclampsia includes the additional symptom of convulsions. The pathophysiology of preeclampsia involves a **generalized arteriolar constriction** that impacts the brain (seizures and stroke), kidneys (oliguria and renal failure), liver (edema), and small blood vessels (thrombocytopenia and disseminated intravascular coagulation). Treatment of severe preeclampsia involves **magnesium sulfate** (for seizure prophylaxis) and **hydralazine** (blood pressure control); once the patient is stabilized, delivery of the fetus should ensue immediately. Risk factors include nulliparity, diabetes, hypertension, renal disease, twin gestation, or hydatidiform mole (produces first-trimester preeclampsia).

II The Placenta as an Endocrine Organ

A. HUMAN CHORIONIC GONADOTROPIN (hCG) is a glycoprotein hormone that stimulates the production of progesterone by the corpus luteum.

B. HUMAN PLACENTAL LACTOGEN (hPL) is a protein hormone that induces lipolysis, elevating free fatty acid levels in the mother; it is considered to be the "growth hormone" of the fetus.

C. ESTRONE, ESTRADIOL (MOST POTENT), AND ESTRIOL are steroid hormones produced by the placenta, but little is known about their specific functions in either the mother or the fetus.

D. PROGESTERONE is a steroid hormone that maintains the endometrium during pregnancy, is used by the fetal adrenal cortex as a precursor for glucocorticoid and mineralocorticoid synthesis, and is used by the fetal testes as a precursor for testosterone synthesis.

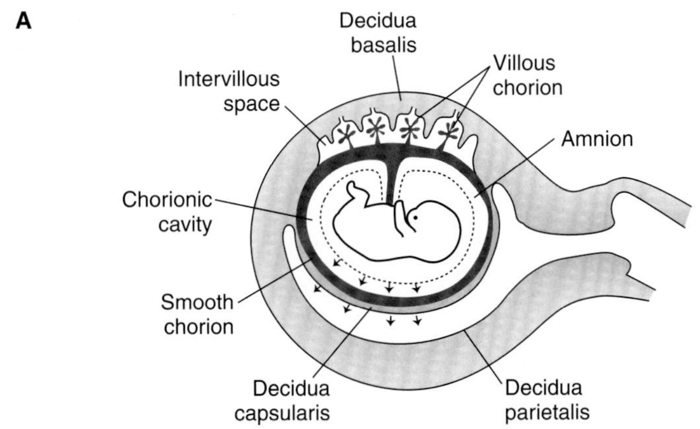

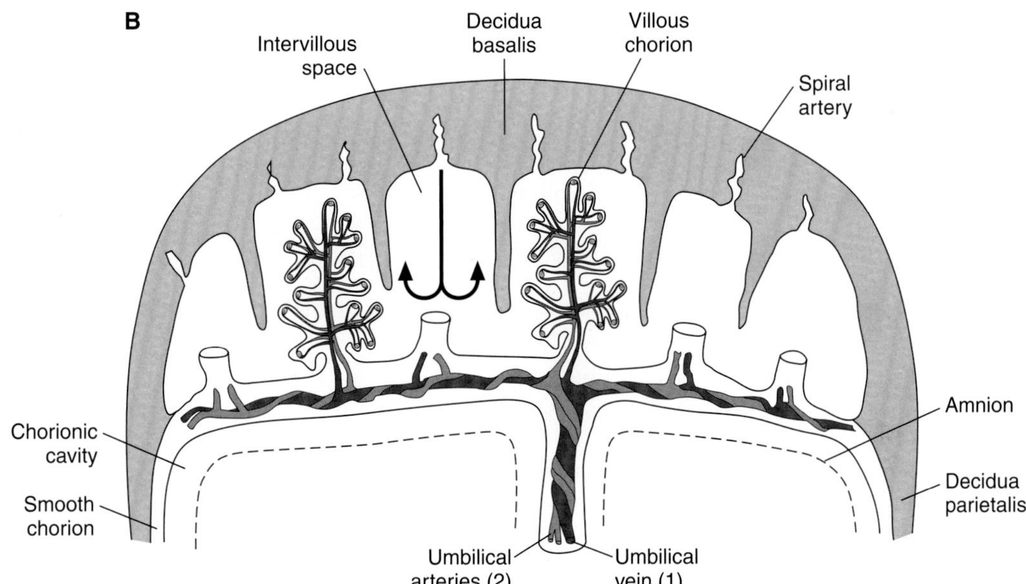

● **Figure 5-1 (A)** Relationship of the fetus, uterus, and placenta in the early fetal period. The small arrows (*outer set*) indicate that as the fetus grows within the uterine wall the decidua capsularis expands and fuses with the decidua parietalis, thereby obliterating the uterine cavity. The small arrows (*inner set*) indicate that as the fetus grows, the amnion expands toward the smooth chorion, thereby obliterating the chorionic cavity. **(B)** Diagram of the placenta. This diagram of the placenta is oriented in the same direction as (A) for comparison. Note the relationship of the villous chorion (fetal component) to the decidua basalis (maternal component). Maternal blood enters the intervillous space (*curved arrow*) via the spiral arteries and bathes the villi in maternal blood. The villi contain fetal capillaries, and thus maternal and fetal blood exchange occurs.

III The Placental Membrane (Table 5-1)

A. In early pregnancy, the placental membrane consists of the **syncytiotrophoblast, cytotrophoblast (Langerhans cells), connective tissue**, and **endothelium of the fetal capillaries. Hofbauer cells** are found in the connective tissue and are most likely macrophages.

TABLE 5-1 **SUBSTANCES THAT CROSS OR DO NOT CROSS THE PLACENTAL MEMBRANE**

Beneficial Substances That Cross the Placental Membrane
O_2, CO_2
Glucose, L-form amino acids, free fatty acids, vitamins
H_2O, Na^+, K^+, Ca^{2+}, Cl^-, I^-, PO_4^{2-}
Urea, uric acid, bilirubin
Fetal and maternal red blood cells
Maternal serum proteins, α-fetoprotein, transferrin–Fe^{2+} complex, low-density lipoprotein, prolactin
Steroid hormones (unconjugated)
Immunoglobulin G, Immunoglobulin A

Harmful Substances That Cross the Placental Membrane
Viruses, e.g., rubella, cytomegalovirus, herpes simplex type 2, varicella zoster, Coxsackie, variola, measles, poliomyelitis
Category X drugs (absolute contraindication in pregnancy), e.g., thalidomide, aminopterin, methotrexate, busulfan (Myleran), chlorambucil (Leukeran), cyclophosphamide (Cytoxan), phenytoin (Dilantin), triazolam (Halcion), estazolam (Prosom), warfarin (Coumadin), isotretinoin (Accutane), clomiphene (Clomid), diethylstilbestrol (DES), ethisterone, norethisterone, megestrol (Megace), oral contraceptives (Ovcon, Levlen, Norinyl), nicotine, alcohol, angiotensin-converting-enzyme inhibitors (Captopril, enalapril)
Category D drugs (definite evidence of risk to fetus), e.g., tetracycline (Achromycin), doxycycline (Vibramycin), streptomycin, amikacin, tobramycin (Nebcin), phenobarbital (Donnatal), pentobarbital (Nembutal), valproic acid (Depakene), diazepam (Valium), chlordiazepoxide (Librium), alprazolam (Xanax), lorazepam (Ativan), lithium, hydrochlorothiazide (Diuril)
Carbon monoxide
Organic mercury, lead, polychlorinated biphenyls (PCBs), potassium iodide, cocaine, heroin
Toxoplasma gondii, Treponema palladium, Listeria monocytogenes
Rubella virus vaccine
Anti-Rh antibodies

Substances That Do Not Cross the Placental Membrane
Maternally derived cholesterol, triglycerides, and phospholipids
Protein hormones (e.g., insulin)
Drugs (e.g., succinylcholine, curare, heparin, methyldopa, drugs similar to amino acids)
Immunoglobulins D, E, M
Bacteria in general

B. In late pregnancy, the cytotrophoblast degenerates, and the connective tissue is displaced by the growth of fetal capillaries, leaving the **syncytiotrophoblast** and the **fetal capillary endothelium.**

C. The **placental membrane** separates maternal blood from fetal blood. A common misperception is that the placental membrane acts as a strict "barrier." However, a wide variety of substances freely cross the placental membrane. Substances that cross can be either beneficial or harmful. Some substances do not cross the placental membrane.

D. CLINICAL CONSIDERATION: ERYTHROBLASTOSIS FETALIS. The **Rh factor** is clinically important in pregnancy. If the mother is Rh-negative and the fetus is Rh-positive, the mother will produce Rh antibodies. This situation will not affect the first pregnancy. In the second pregnancy with an Rh-positive fetus, a hemolytic condition of red blood cells (RBCs) occurs, known as **Rh-hemolytic disease of newborn (erythroblastosis fetalis)**. This causes destruction of fetal RBCs, which leads to the release of large amounts of **unconjugated bilirubin** (a breakdown product of hemoglobin). This causes fetal brain damage due to a condition called **kernicterus**, which is a pathological deposition of bilirubin in the basal ganglia. **Ultraviolet (UV) light** is used to treat the newborn with physiological jaundice. **Severe hemolytic disease**, in which the fetus is severely anemic and demonstrates total body edema (i.e., **hydrops fetalis**), may lead to death. In these cases, an intrauterine transfusion is indicated. **Rh_0(D) immune globulin (RhoGAM, MICRhoGAM)** is a human immunoglobulin G (IgG) preparation that contains antibodies against Rh factor and prevents a maternal antibody response to Rh-positive cells that may enter the maternal bloodstream of an Rh-negative mother. This drug is administered to Rh-negative mothers during the third trimester and within 72 hours after the birth of an Rh-positive baby to prevent erythroblastosis fetalis during subsequent pregnancies.

IV Amniotic Fluid

Amniotic Fluid is maternally derived water that contains: electrolytes, carbohydrates, amino acids, lipids, proteins (hormones, enzymes, α-fetoprotein), urea, creatinine, lactate, pyruvate, desquamated fetal cells, fetal urine, fetal feces (meconium), and fetal lung liquid (useful for lecithin/sphingomyelin [L/S] ratio measurement for lung maturity).

A. PRODUCTION OF AMNIOTIC FLUID

1. Amniotic fluid is constantly produced during pregnancy by the following: **direct transfer** from maternal circulation in response to osmotic and hydrostatic forces and **excretion of fetal urine by the kidneys** into the amniotic sac. Kidney defects (e.g., bilateral kidney agenesis) result in **oligohydramnios**.

B. RESORPTION OF AMNIOTIC FLUID

1. Amniotic fluid is constantly resorbed during pregnancy by the following sequence of events: The fetus swallows amniotic fluid, amniotic fluid is absorbed into fetal blood through the gastrointestinal tract, and excess amniotic fluid is removed via the placenta and passed into maternal blood. Swallowing defects (e.g., esophageal atresia) or absorption defects (e.g., duodenal atresia) result in **polyhydramnios**.

C. THE AMOUNT OF AMNIOTIC FLUID

1. Is gradually increased during pregnancy from **50 mL at week 12** to **1000 mL at term**. The rate of water exchange within the amniotic sac at term is 400–500 mL/hr, with a net flow of 125–200 mL/hr moving from the amniotic fluid into the maternal blood. The near-term fetus excretes about 500 mL of urine daily, which is mostly water because the placenta exchanges metabolic wastes. The fetus swallows about 400 mL of amniotic fluid daily.

D. CLINICAL CONSIDERATIONS

1. **Oligohydramnios** occurs when there is a low amount of amniotic fluid (**<400 mL in late pregnancy**). Oligohydramnios may be associated with the inability of the fetus to excrete urine into the amniotic sac due to **renal agenesis**. This results in many fetal deformities (**Potter syndrome**) and **hypoplastic lungs** due to increased pressure on the fetal thorax.
2. **Polyhydramnios** occurs when there is a high amount of amniotic fluid (**>2000 mL in late pregnancy**). Polyhydramnios may be associated with the inability of the fetus to swallow due to **anencephaly**, **tracheoesophageal fistula**, or **esophageal atresia**. Polyhydramnios is commonly associated with **maternal diabetes**.
3. **α-Fetoprotein (AFP)** is "fetal albumin" that is produced by fetal hepatocytes. AFP is routinely assayed in amniotic fluid and maternal serum between **weeks 14 and 18** of gestation. AFP levels change with gestational age, so that proper interpretation of AFP levels is dependent on an accurate gestational age. Elevated AFP

levels are associated with **neural tube defects** (e.g., **spina bifida or anencephaly**), **omphalocele** (allows fetal serum to leak into the amniotic fluid), and **esophageal and duodenal atresia** (which interfere with fetal swallowing). Reduced AFP levels are associated with **Down syndrome.**

4. **Premature rupture of the amniochorionic membrane** is the most common cause of premature labor and oligohydramnios. It is commonly referred to as "breaking of the water bag."
5. **Amniotic band syndrome** occurs when bands of amniotic membrane encircle and constrict parts of the fetus, causing **limb amputations** and **craniofacial anomalies.**

V Umbilical Cord

A. DESCRIPTION

1. A patent opening called the **primitive umbilical ring** exists on the ventral surface of the developing embryo through which three structures pass: the **yolk sac (vitelline duct)**, **connecting stalk**, and **allantois.** The allantois is not functional in humans and degenerates to form the **median umbilical ligament** in the adult.
2. As the amnion expands, it pushes the vitelline duct, connecting stalk, and allantois together to form the **primitive umbilical cord.**
3. The definitive umbilical cord at term is pearl-white, 1–2 cm in diameter, 50–60 cm long, eccentrically positioned, and contains the **right and left umbilical arteries**, **left umbilical vein**, and **mucus connective tissue (Wharton's jelly).**
4. The right and left umbilical arteries carry deoxygenated blood from the fetus to the placenta. The left umbilical vein carries oxygenated blood from the placenta to the fetus.

B. CLINICAL CONSIDERATIONS

1. **Presence of one umbilical artery** within the umbilical cord is an abnormal finding that suggests cardiovascular abnormalities. Normally, two umbilical arteries are present.
2. **Physical inspection of the umbilicus** in a newborn infant may reveal:
   a. A light-gray, shiny sac indicating an **omphalocele** (see Chapter 7).
   b. A fecal (meconium) discharge indicating a **vitelline fistula** (see Chapter 7).
   c. A urine discharge indicating an **urachal fistula** (see Chapter 8).

VI Vasculogenesis (de novo blood vessel formation) occurs in two general locations as follows.

A. IN EXTRAEMBRYONIC MESODERM. Vasculogenesis occurs first within extraembryonic visceral mesoderm around the yolk sac on day 17. By day 21, vasculogenesis extends into extraembryonic somatic mesoderm located around the connecting stalk to form the **umbilical vessels** and in secondary villi to form **tertiary chorionic villi.** Vasculogenesis occurs by a process in which extraembryonic mesoderm differentiates into **angioblasts**, which form clusters known as **angiogenic cell clusters.** The angioblasts located at the periphery of angiogenic cell clusters give rise to **endothelial cells**, which fuse with each other to form small blood vessels.

B. IN INTRAEMBRYONIC MESODERM. Blood vessels form within the embryo by the same mechanism as in extraembryonic mesoderm. Eventually blood vessels formed in the extraembryonic mesoderm become continuous with blood vessels within the embryo, thereby establishing a blood vascular system between the embryo and the placenta.

VII Hematopoiesis (Figure 5-2).

Hematopoiesis (**blood cell formation**) first occurs within the extraembryonic visceral mesoderm around the yolk sac during week 3 of development. During this process, angioblasts within the center of angiogenic cell clusters give rise to primitive blood cells. Beginning at week 5, hematopoiesis is taken over by a sequence of embryonic organs: **liver, spleen, thymus**, and **bone marrow**.

A. TYPES OF HEMOGLOBIN PRODUCED DURING HEMATOPOIESIS

1. During the period of yolk sac hematopoiesis, the earliest **embryonic form** of hemoglobin, called **hemoglobin $\zeta_2\varepsilon_2$**, is synthesized.
2. During the period of liver hematopoiesis, the **fetal form** of hemoglobin (HbF), called **hemoglobin $\alpha_2\gamma_2$**, is synthesized. **Hemoglobin $\alpha_2\gamma_2$** is the predominant form of hemoglobin during pregnancy because it has a higher affinity for oxygen than the **adult form** of hemoglobin (HbA; **hemoglobin $\alpha_2\beta_2$**) and therefore "pulls" oxygen from the maternal blood into fetal blood.
3. During the period of bone marrow hematopoiesis (about week 30), the **adult form** of hemoglobin, called **hemoglobin $\alpha_2\beta_2$**, is synthesized and gradually replaces **hemoglobin $\alpha_2\gamma_2$**.

B. CLINICAL CONSIDERATIONS

1. **Thalassemia syndromes** are a heterogeneous group of genetic defects characterized by the lack or decreased synthesis of either the α-globin chain (**α-thalassemia**) or β-globin chain (**β-thalassemia**) of hemoglobin $\alpha_2\beta_2$.
   a. **Hydrops fetalis** is the most severe form of α-thalassemia and causes severe pallor, generalized edema, and massive hepatosplenomegaly and invariably leads to intrauterine fetal death.
   b. **β-Thalassemia major (Cooley anemia)** is the most severe form of β-thalassemia and causes a severe, transfusion-dependent anemia. It is most common in Mediterranean countries and parts of Africa and Southeast Asia.
2. **Hydroxyurea** (a cytotoxic drug) has been shown to promote HbF production by the reactivation of γ-chain synthesis. Hydroxyurea has been especially useful in the treatment of **sickle cell disease**, in which the presence of HbF counteracts the low oxygen affinity of sickle Hb (HbS) and inhibits the sickling process.

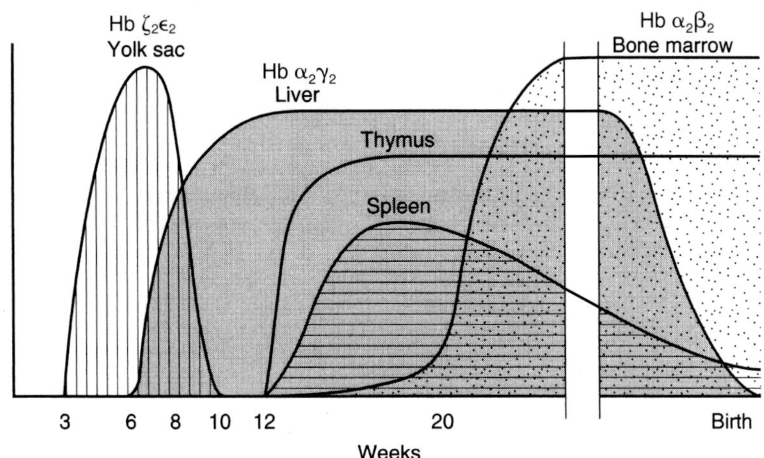

● **Figure 5-2** Diagram showing the contribution of various organs to hematopoiesis during embryonic and fetal development. Hb = hemoglobin.

Fetal Circulation (Figure 5-3). **Fetal circulation involves three shunts: the** ductus venosus, ductus arteriosus, **and** foramen ovale.

A. Highly oxygenated and nutrient-enriched blood returns to the fetus from the placenta via the **left umbilical vein**. (Note: Highly oxygenated blood is carried by the left umbilical vein, not by an artery as in the adult.) Some blood percolates through the hepatic

Shunts
③ Ductus arteriosus
(*Adult remnant:* ligamentum arteriosum)
② Foramen ovale
(*Adult remnant:* fossa ovale)
Inferior vena cava
Liver
Left umbilical vein (↑O_2)
(*Adult remnant:* ligamentum teres)
① Ductus venosus
(*Adult remnant:* ligamentum venosum)
Right and left umbilical arteries (↓O_2)
(*Adult remnant:* medial umbilical ligaments)

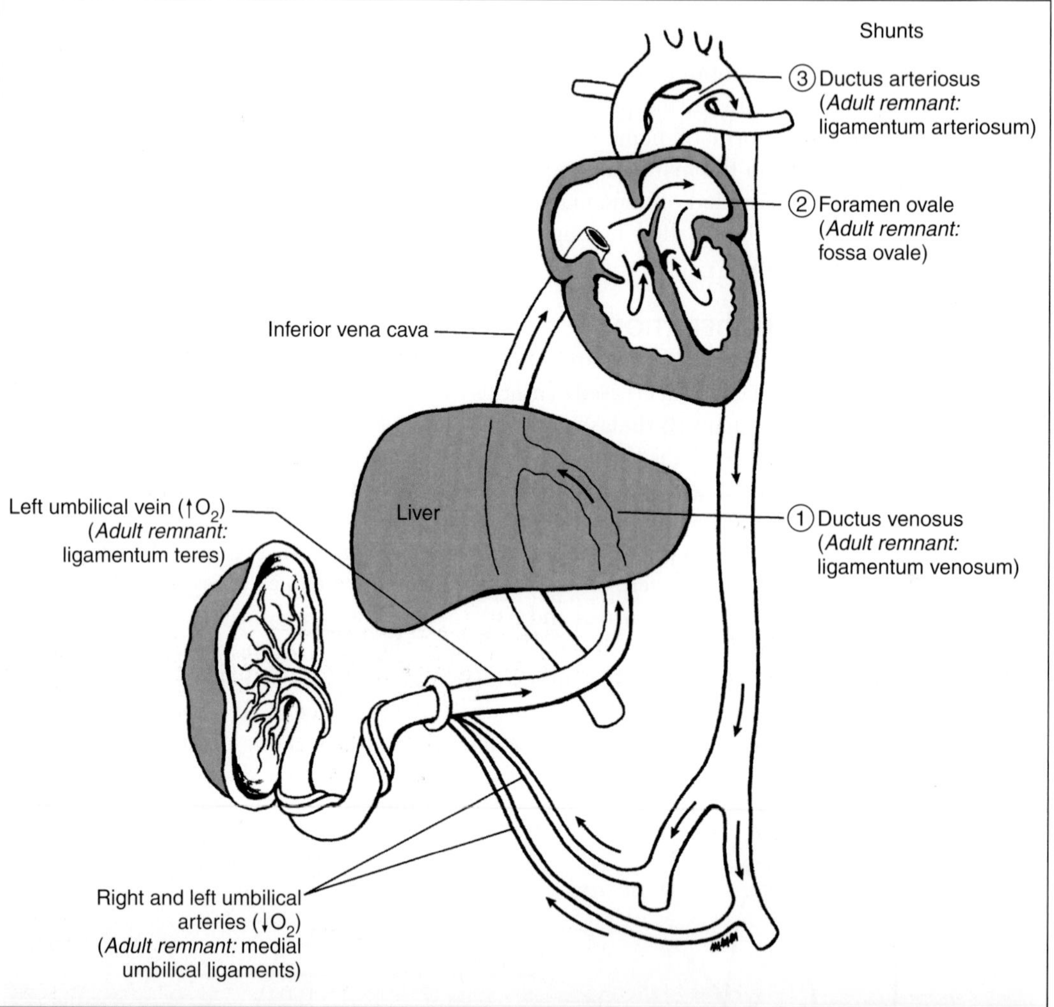

Remants Created by Closure of Fetal Circulatory Structures

Fetal Structure	Adult Remnant
Right and left umbilical arteries	Medial umbilical ligaments
Left umbilical vein	Ligamentum teres
Ductus venosus	Ligamentum venosum
Foramen ovale	Fossa ovale
Ductus arteriosus	Ligamentum arteriosum

● **Figure 5-3 Fetal circulation.** Note the three shunts and the changes that occur after birth (remnants).

sinusoids; most of the blood bypasses the sinusoids by passing through the **ductus venosus** and enters the inferior vena cava (IVC). From the IVC, blood enters the right atrium, where most of the blood bypasses the right ventricle through the **foramen ovale** to enter the left atrium. From the left atrium, blood enters the left ventricle and is delivered to fetal tissues via the aorta.

B. Poorly oxygenated and nutrient-poor fetal blood is sent back to the placenta via **right and left umbilical arteries.**

C. Some blood in the right atrium enters the right ventricle; blood in the right ventricle enters the pulmonary trunk, but most of the blood bypasses the lungs through the **ductus arteriosus**. Fetal lungs receive only a minimal amount of blood for growth and development; the blood is returned to the left ventricle via pulmonary veins. Fetal lungs are not capable of performing their adult respiratory function because they are functionally immature and the fetus is underwater (amnionic fluid). The placenta provides respiratory function.

D. Circulatory system changes at birth are facilitated by a **decrease in right atrial pressure** from occlusion of placental circulation and by an **increase in left atrial pressure** due to increased pulmonary venous return. Changes include closure of the right and left umbilical arteries, left umbilical vein, ductus venosus, ductus arteriosus, and foramen ovale.

Case Study 1

A 37-year-old woman who is in her third trimester comes into your clinic complaining of bleeding that lasted for about "an hour or two." She remarks she noticed that the bleeding was "very bright red" in color but felt no noticeable pain. She says that she did nothing to cause the bleeding and "was concerned for the safety of her baby." What is the most likely diagnosis?

Differentials

- Placenta previa, placental abruption, placenta accreta

Relevant Physical Exam Findings

- No abdominal or pelvic pain could be found on palpation

Relevant Lab Findings

- Transvaginal ultrasound shows an intact, normally implanted placenta. However, the placenta was located in close proximity to the internal os.

Diagnosis

- **Placenta previa:** This is a classic case of placenta previa. The patient is in advancing maternal age and shows bright-red bleeding during the third trimester with the implantation located at or near the internal os. Placental abruption would have shown a separation of the placenta and showed dark-red bleeding accompanied by abdominal pain. Placenta accreta would have shown the placenta implanted much deeper in the myometrium.

Case Study 2

A 34-year-old woman who is in her third trimester complains of her hands and face "swelling up a few days ago." She remarks that she has also felt like "her heart was racing a mile a minute." What is the most likely diagnosis?

Differentials

- Preeclampsia, renal disease, molar pregnancy

Relevant Physical Exam Findings

- Hypertension
- Hand and facial edema

Relevant Lab Findings

- Proteinuria
- Ultrasound was unremarkable

Diagnosis

- Preeclampsia: Her symptoms of hypertension, proteinuria, and edema are all telltale signs of preeclampsia. In addition, her advancing age has left her susceptible to this condition. Molar pregnancy is normally seen in the first trimester. Renal disease is unlikely because there were no findings other than proteinuria.

Chapter **6**

Cardiovascular System

I **Formation of Heart Tube.** Lateral plate mesoderm (at the cephalic area of the embryo) will split into a somatic layer and a splanchnic layer, thus forming the **pericardial cavity**. Precardiac mesoderm is preferentially distributed to the splanchnic layer and is now called **heart-forming regions (HFRs)**. As lateral folding of the embryo occurs, the HFRs will fuse in the midline to form a continuous sheet of mesoderm. Hypertrophied foregut endoderm secretes **vascular endothelial growth factor (VEGF)**, which induces the sheet of mesoderm to form discontinuous vascular channels that eventually get remodeled into a single **endocardial tube (endocardium)**. Mesoderm around the endocardium forms the myocardium, which secretes a layer of extracellular matrix proteins called **cardiac jelly**. Mesoderm migrating into the cardiac region from the coelomic wall near the liver forms the **epicardium**.

II **Primitive Heart Tube Dilatations (Figure 6-1).** Five dilatations soon become apparent along the length of the tube: the **truncus arteriosus**, **bulbus cordis**, **primitive ventricle**, **primitive atrium**, and **sinus venosus**. These five dilatations develop into the adult structures of the heart.

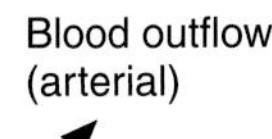

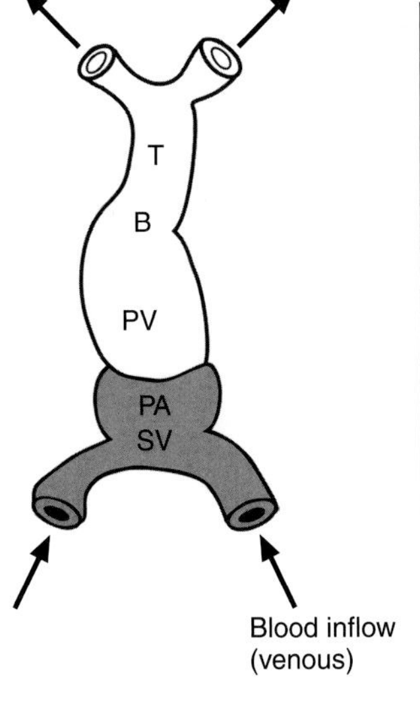

Embryonic Dilatation	Adult Structure
Truncus arteriosus (T)	Aorta Pulmonary trunk
Bulbus cordis (B)	Smooth part of right ventricle **(conus arteriosus)** Smooth part of left ventricle **(aortic vestibule)**
Primitive ventricle (PV)	Trabeculated part of right ventricle Trabeculated part of left ventricle
Primitive atrium (PA)	Trabeculated part of right atrium Trabeculated part of left atrium
Sinus venosus (SV)	Smooth part of right atrium **(sinus venarum)*** Coronary sinus Oblique vein of left atrium

*The smooth part of the left atrium is formed by incorporation of parts of the **pulmonary veins** into the atrial wall. The junction of the trabeculated and smooth parts of the right atrium is called the **crista terminalis.**

● **Figure 6-1 The five dilatations of the heart tube.** B = bulbus cordis, PA = primitive atrium, PV = primitive ventricle, SV = sinus venosus, T = truncus arteriosus. White area: arterial portion. Shaded area: venous portion.

III The Aorticopulmonary (AP) Septum (Figure 6-2)

A. FORMATION (FIGURE 6-2A). **Neural crest** cells migrate from the hindbrain region through pharyngeal arches 3, 4, and 6 and invade both the **truncal ridges and the bulbar ridges**. **The truncal** and bulbar ridges grow and twist around each other in a spiral fashion and eventually fuse to form the AP septum. The AP septum divides the truncus arteriosus and bulbus cordis into the aorta and pulmonary trunk.

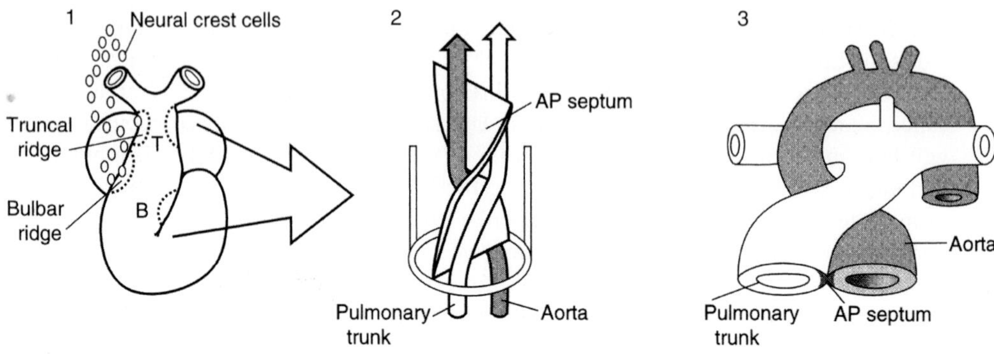

● **Figure 6-2A Formation of the aorticopulmonary (AP) septum (1–3).**

B. CLINICAL CONSIDERATIONS

1. **Persistent truncus arteriosus (PTA)** is caused by abnormal neural crest cell migration such that there is only *partial* development of the AP septum (Figure 6-2B). PTA results in a condition in which one large vessel leaves the heart and receives blood from both the right and the left ventricles. PTA is usually accompanied by a membranous ventricular septal defect (VSD) and is associated clinically with **marked cyanosis (right-to-left [R → L] shunting of blood)**.

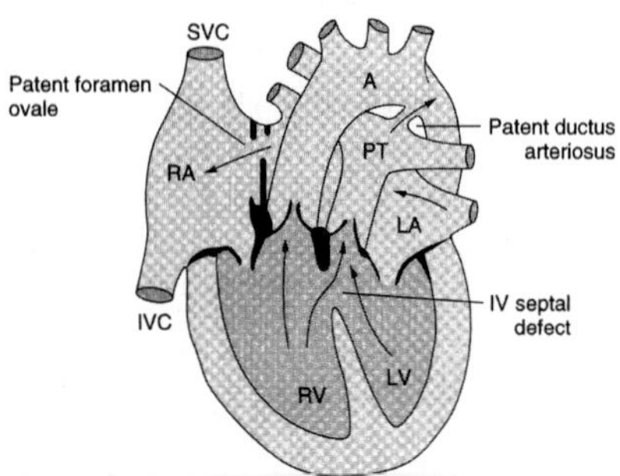

● **Figure 6-2B Aorticopulmonary septal defects: persistent truncus arteriosus.** Arrows indicate the direction of blood flow. A = aorta; IVC = inferior vena cava; LA = left atrium; LV = left ventricle; RA = right atrium; RV = right ventricle; PT = pulmonary trunk; SVC = superior vena cava.

2. **D-transposition of the great arteries (complete)** is caused by abnormal neural crest cell migration such that there is *nonspiral* development of the AP septum (Figure 6-2C). D-transposition results in a condition in which the aorta arises abnormally from the right ventricle and the pulmonary trunk arises abnormally from the left ventricle; hence the systemic and pulmonary circulations are *completely* separated from each other. It is incompatible with life unless an accompanying shunt exists like a VSD, patent foramen ovale, or *patent ductus* arteriosus. It is associated clinically with **marked cyanosis (R → L shunting of blood)**.
3. **L-transposition of the great vessels (corrected)** (Figure 6-2D). In L-transposition, the aorta and pulmonary trunk are transposed and the ventricles are "inverted" such that the anatomical right ventricle lies on the left side and the anatomical left ventricle lies on the right side. These two major deviations offset one another such that blood flow pattern is normal.
4. **Tetralogy of Fallot (TF) is caused by an abnormal neural crest cell migration such that there is** *skewed* development of the AP septum (Figure 6-2E). TF results in a condition in which the *pul*monary trunk obtains a small diameter while the aorta obtains a large diameter. TF is characterized by four classic malformations: **pulmonary stenosis, right ventricular hypertrophy, overriding aorta, and ventricular septal defect** (note the mnemonic **PROVE**). TF is associated clinically with **marked cyanosis (R → L shunting of blood)** in which the clinical consequences depend primarily on the severity of the pulmonary stenosis.

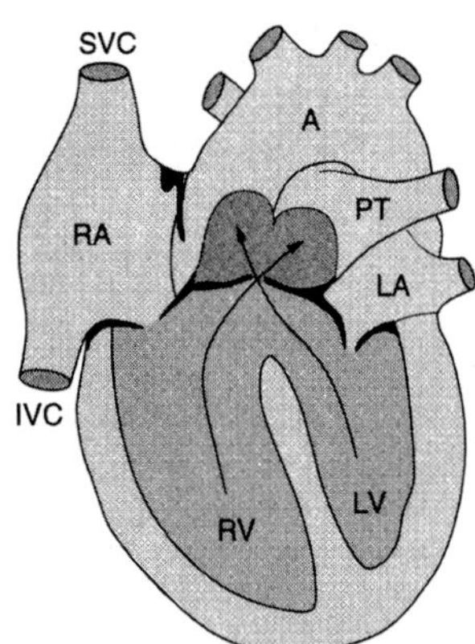

● **Figure 6-2C Aorticopulmonary septal defects: D-transposition of the great arteries (complete).** IV = interventricular; see legend to Figure 6-2B for other abbreviations.

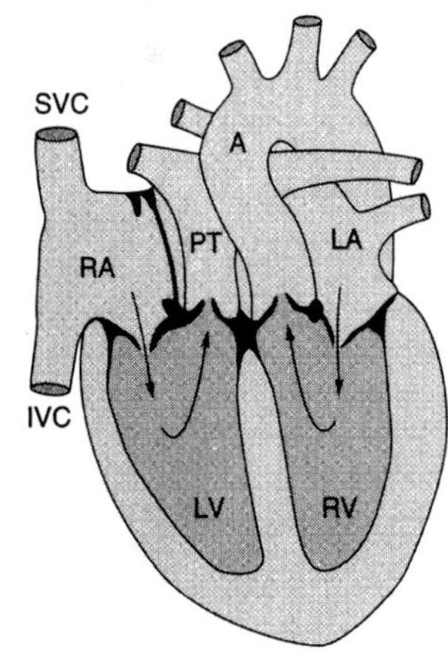

● **Figure 6-2D Aorticopulmonary septal defects: L-transposition of the great arteries.** See legend to Figure 6-2B for abbreviations.

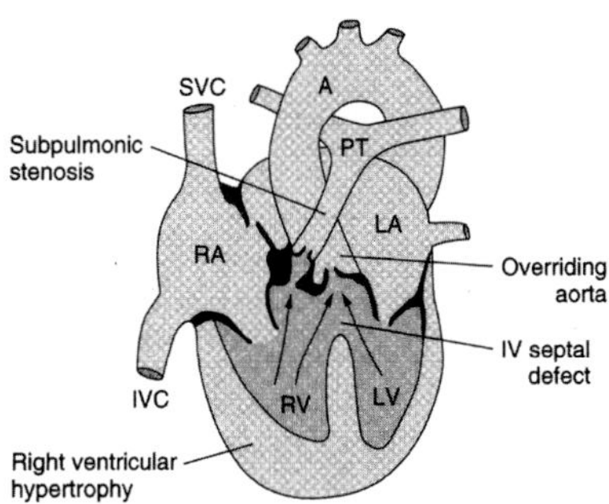

● **Figure 6-2E Aorticopulmonary septal defects: tetralogy of Fallot.** IV = interventricular; see legend to Figure 6-2B for other abbreviations.

IV The Atrial Septum (Figure 6-3)

A. FORMATION (FIGURE 6-3A). The crescent-shaped **septum primum** forms in the roof of the primitive atrium and grows toward the atrioventricular (AV) cushions in the AV canal. The **foramen primum** forms between the free edge of the septum primum and the AV cushions; it is closed when the septum primum fuses with the AV cushions. The **foramen secundum** forms in the center of the septum primum. The crescent-shaped septum secundum forms to the right of the septum primum. The **foramen ovale** is the opening between the upper and the lower limbs of the septum secundum. During embryonic life, blood is shunted from the right atrium to the left atrium via the foramen ovale. Immediately after birth, functional closure of the foramen ovale is facilitated both by a **decrease in right atrial pressure** from occlusion of placental circulation and by an **increase in left atrial pressure** due to increased pulmonary venous return. Later in life, the septum primum and septum secundum anatomically fuse to complete the formation of the atrial septum.

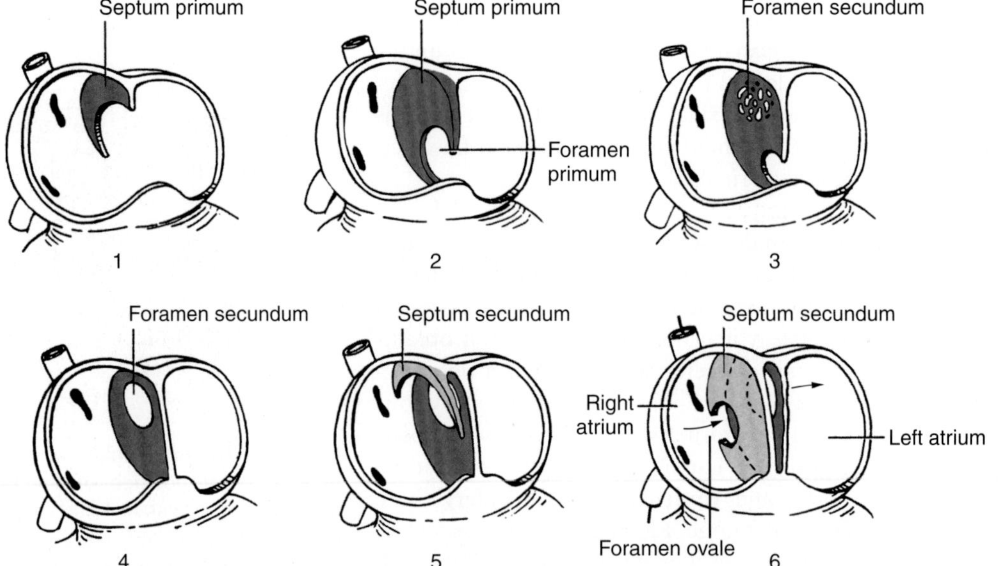

● **Figure 6-3A Formation of the atrial septum (1–6).** The arrows in 6 indicate the direction of blood flow across the fully developed septum, from the right atrium to the left atrium.

B. CLINICAL CONSIDERATIONS. Atrial septal defects (ASDs) are noted on auscultation with a loud S1 and a wide, fixed, split S2 and are characterized by L → R shunting of blood.

1. **Foramen secundum defect** is caused by excessive resorption of septum primum, septum secundum, or both (Figure 6-3B). This results in a condition in which there is an opening between the right and the left atria. Some defects can be tolerated for a long time, with clinical symptoms manifesting as late as age 30 years. It is the most common clinically significant ASD.
2. **Common atrium (cor triloculare biventriculare)** is caused by the complete failure of septum primum and septum secundum to develop (Figure 6-3C). This results in a condition in which there is formation of only one atrium.
3. **Probe patency of the foramen ovale** is caused by incomplete anatomic fusion of septum primum and septum secundum. It is present in approximately 25% of the population and is usually of no clinical importance.
4. **Premature closure of foramen ovale** is closure of foramen ovale during prenatal life. It results in hypertrophy of the right side of the heart and underdevelopment of the left side of the heart.

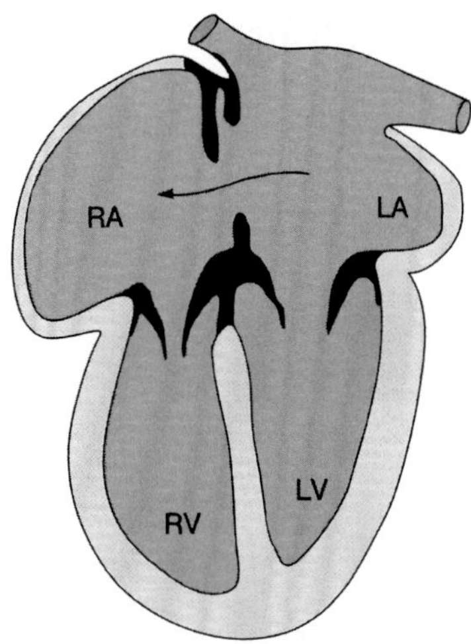

● **Figure 6-3B Atrial septal defects (ASDs): foramen secundum defect.** LA = left atrium; LV = left ventricle; RA = right atrium; RV = right ventricle.

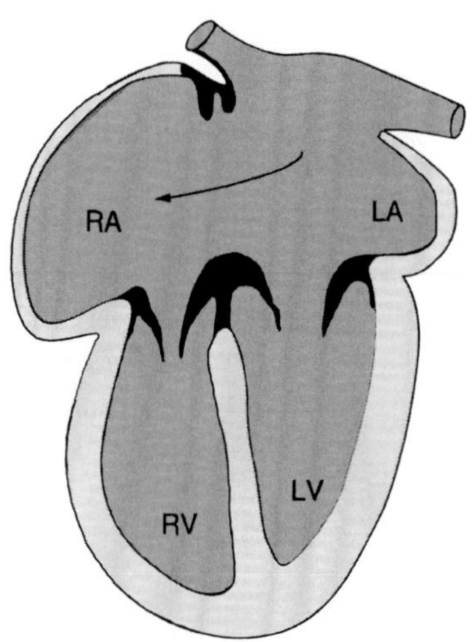

● **Figure 6-3C Atrial septal defects: common atrium.** LA = left atrium; LV = left ventricle; RA = right atrium; RV = right ventricle.

V The Atrioventricular (AV) Septum (Figure 6-4)

A. FORMATION (FIGURE 6-4A). The **dorsal AV cushion** and **ventral AV cushion** approach each other and fuse to form the AV septum. The AV septum partitions the AV canal into the right AV canal and the left AV canal.

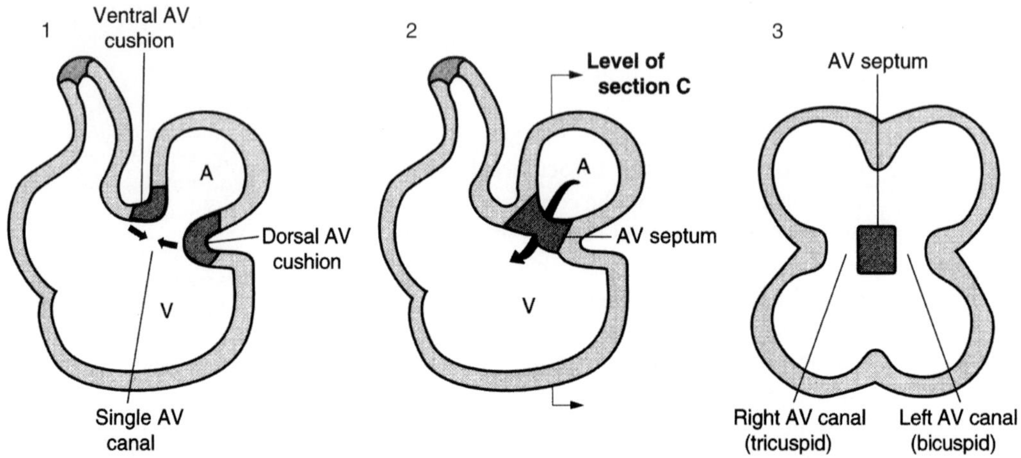

● **Figure 6-4A Formation of the atrioventricular (AV) septum (1–3), which partitions the atrioventricular canal.** A = atrium; V = ventricle.

B. CLINICAL CONSIDERATIONS

1. **Persistent common AV canal** is caused by failure of fusion of the dorsal and ventral AV cushions (Figure 6-4B). It results in a condition in which the common AV canal is never partitioned into the right and left AV canals, so that a large hole can be found in the center of the heart. Consequently, the tricuspid and bicuspid valves are represented by one valve common to both sides of the heart. Two common hemodynamic abnormalities are found:
   a. L → R shunting of blood from the left atrium to the right atrium, causing an enlarged right atrium and right ventricle.
   b. Mitral valve regurgitation, causing an enlarged left atrium and left ventricle.

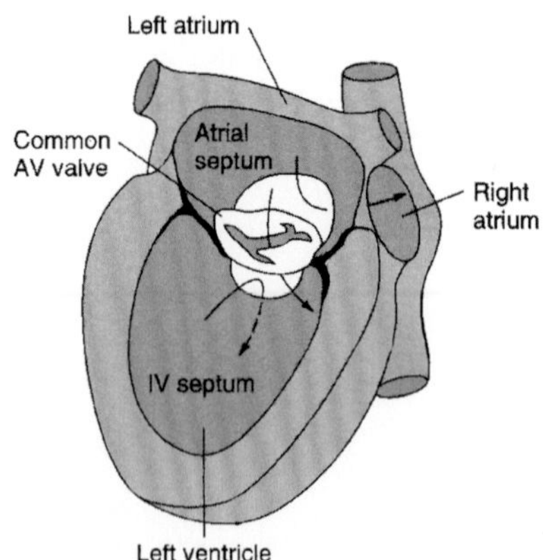

● **Figure 6-4B Atrioventricular (AV) septal defects: persistent common AV canal.** IV = interventricular.

2. **Ebstein's anomaly** is caused by the failure of the posterior and septal leaflets of the tricuspid valve to attach normally to the annulus fibrosus; instead they are displaced inferiorly into the right ventricle (Figure 6-4C). It results in a condition in which the right ventricle is divided into a large, upper, "atrialized" portion and a small, lower, functional portion. Due to the small, functional portion of the right ventricle, there is reduced amount of blood available to the pulmonary trunk. It is usually associated with an ASD. The anteroposterior radiograph shows massive cardiomegaly due to enlargement of the right atrium.
3. **Foramen primum defect** is caused by a failure of the AV septum to fuse with septum primum (Figure 6-4D). It results in a condition in which the foramen primum is never closed and is generally accompanied by an abnormal mitral valve.
4. **Tricuspid atresia (hypoplastic right heart)** is caused by an insufficient amount of AV cushion tissue available for the formation of the tricuspid valve (Figure 6-4E). It results in a condition in which there is complete agenesis of the tricuspid valve so that no communication between the right atrium and the right ventricle exists. It is associated clinically with **marked cyanosis** and is always accompanied by the following: patent foramen ovale, interventricular septum defect, overdeveloped left ventricle, and underdeveloped right ventricle. The anteroposterior radiograph shows a normal-sized heart with a convex left cardiac contour.

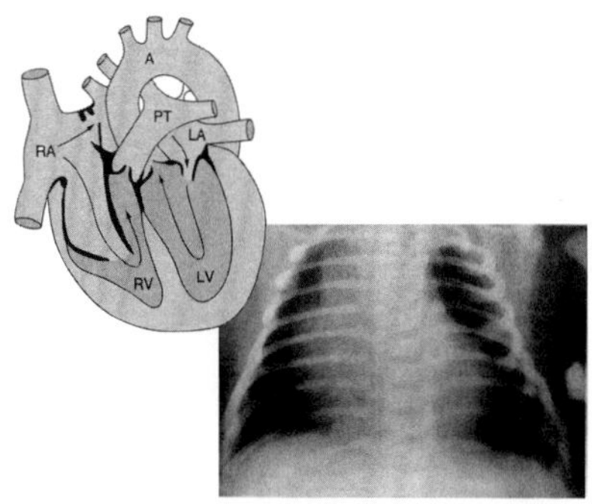

● **Figure 6-4C Atrioventricular septal defects: Ebstein's anomaly.** A = aorta; LA = left atrium; LV = left ventricle; RA = right atrium; RV = right ventricle; PT = pulmonary trunk.

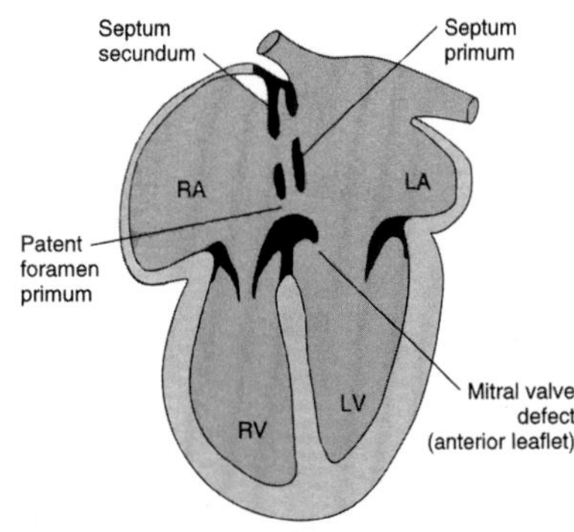

● **Figure 6-4D Atrioventricular septal defects: foramen primum defect.** LA = left atrium; LV = left ventricle; RA = right atrium; RV = right ventricle.

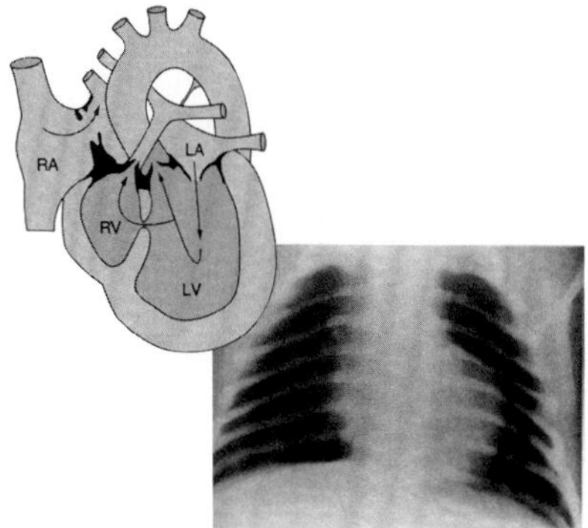

● **Figure 6-4E Atrioventricular septal defects: tricuspid atresia.** LA = left atrium; LV = left ventricle; RA = right atrium; RV = right ventricle.

The Interventricular (IV) Septum (Figure 6-5)

A. FORMATION (FIGURE 6-5A). THE MUSCULAR IV septum develops in the midline on the floor of the primitive ventricle and grows toward the fused AV cushions. The IV foramen is located between the free edge of the muscular IV septum and the fused AV cushions. This foramen is closed by the membranous IV septum, which forms by the proliferation and fusion of tissue from three sources: the right bulbar ridge, the left bulbar ridge, and the AV cushions.

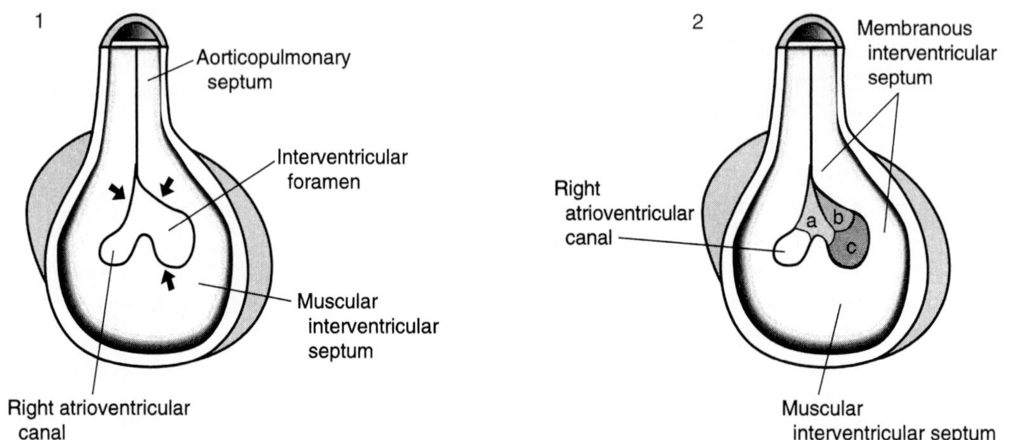

● Figure 6-5A Formation of the interventricular (IV) septum (1,2), which partitions the primitive ventricle. Shaded portion (a, b, c) in 2 indicates the three sources of the membranous interventricular septum. a = right bulbar ridge; b = left bulbar ridge; c = atrioventricular cushions.

B. CLINICAL CONSIDERATIONS. IV SEPTAL DEFECTS (VSDS)

1. **Membranous VSD** is caused by faulty fusion of the **right bulbar ridge**, the **left bulbar ridge**, and the **AV cushions** (**Figure 6-5B**). It results in a condition in which an opening between the right and left ventricles allows free flow of blood. A large VSD is initially associated with L → R shunting of blood, increased pulmonary blood flow, and pulmonary hypertension. Patients with L → R shunting of blood complain of **excessive fatigue on exertion**. The anteroposterior radiograph demonstrates cardiomegaly and a marked enlargement of the main pulmonary artery (arrow in Figure 6-5B).

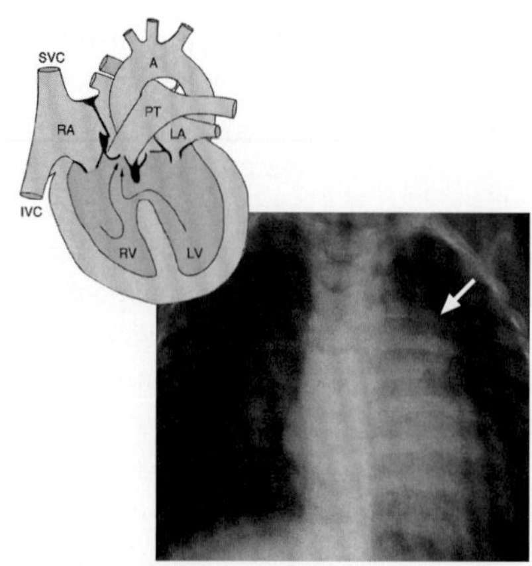

● Figure 6-5B Interventricular septal defects (VSDs): membranous VSD. A = aorta; IVC = inferior vena cava; LA = left atrium; LV = left ventricle; RA = right atrium; RV = right ventricle; PT = pulmonary trunk; SVC = superior vena cava.

2. **Eisenmenger syndrome (uncorrected VSD, ASD, or PDA).** Initially, a VSD, ASD, or PDA is associated with L → R shunting of blood, increased pulmonary blood flow, and pulmonary hypertension. Later, the pulmonary hypertension causes marked proliferation of the tunica intima and tunica media of pulmonary muscular arteries and arterioles, resulting in a narrowing of their lumen. Ultimately, pulmonary resistance may become higher than systemic resistance and cause **R → L shunting** of blood and **cyanosis**.
3. **Muscular VSD** is caused by single or multiple perforations in the muscular IV septum.
4. **Common ventricle (cor triloculare biatriatum)** is caused by failure of the membranous and muscular IV septa to form.

VII Development of the Arterial System (Table 6-1)

A. FORMATION. In the head and neck region, the arterial pattern develops mainly from six pairs of arteries (called **aortic arches**) that course through the pharyngeal arches. The aortic arch arteries undergo a complex remodeling process that results in the adult arterial pattern. In the rest of the body, the arterial patterns develop mainly from the **right and left dorsal aortae**. The right and left dorsal aortae fuse to form the **dorsal aorta**, which then sprouts **posterolateral arteries**, **lateral arteries**, and **ventral arteries (vitelline and umbilical)**.

B. CLINICAL CONSIDERATIONS

1. **Postductal coarctation** of the aorta occurs when the aorta is abnormally constricted. A postductal coarctation is found distal to the origin of the left subclavian artery and inferior to the ductus arteriosus. It is clinically associated with increased blood pressure in the upper extremities, lack of pulse in femoral artery, high risk of both cerebral hemorrhage, and bacterial endocarditis. Collateral circulation around the constriction involves the internal thoracic, intercostal, superior epigastric, inferior epigastric, and external iliac arteries. Dilation of the intercostal arteries causes erosion of the lower border of the ribs (called "rib notching"), which can be seen on X-ray. Less commonly, a **preductal coarctation** may occur where the constriction is located superior to the ductus arteriosus. Turner syndrome (45, XO) is associated with a preductal coarctation.
2. **Patent ductus arteriosus (PDA)** occurs when the ductus arteriosus—a connection between the left pulmonary artery and aorta—fails to close. Normally the ductus arteriosus functionally closes within a few hours after birth via smooth muscle contraction to ultimately form the **ligamentum arteriosum**. A PDA causes L → R shunting **of oxygen-rich blood** from the aorta back into the pulmonary circulation. A PDA can be treated with prostaglandin-synthesis inhibitors (such as indomethacin), acetylcholine, histamine, and catecholamines, all of which promote closure of the ductus arteriosus. Prostaglandin E (PGE_1), intrauterine asphyxia, and neonatal asphyxia sustain patency of the ductus arteriosus. A PDA is very common in premature infants and maternal rubella infection.

VIII Development of the Venous System (Table 6-1).

The venous system develops from the **vitelline**, **umbilical**, and **cardinal veins** that empty into the sinus venosus. These veins undergo remodeling due to a redirection of venous blood from the left side of the body to the right side in order to empty into the right atrium.

TABLE 6-1 DEVELOPMENT OF THE ARTERIAL AND VENOUS SYSTEM

Embryonic Structure	Adult Structure
Aortic Arches	
1	Maxillary artery (portion of)
2	Stapedial artery (portion of)
3	Right and left common carotid arteries (portion of) Right and left internal carotid arteries
4	Right subclavian artery (portion of) Arch of the aorta (portion of)
5	Regresses in the human
6[a]	Right and left pulmonary arteries (portion of) Ductus arteriosus
Dorsal Aorta	
Posterolateral branches	Arteries to upper and lower extremity, intercostal, lumbar, and lateral sacral arteries
Lateral branches	Renal, suprarenal, and gonadal arteries
Ventral branches	
Vitelline arteries	Celiac, superior mesenteric, and inferior mesenteric arteries
Umbilical arteries	Internal iliac arteries (portion of), superior vesical arteries, medial umbilical ligaments
Vitelline Veins	
Right and Left	Portion of the IVC,[b] hepatic veins and sinusoids, ductus venosus, portal vein, inferior mesenteric vein, superior mesenteric vein, splenic vein
Umbilical Veins	
Right	Hepatic sinusoids (degenerates early in fetal life)
Left	Hepatic sinusoids, ligamentum teres
Cardinal Veins	
Anterior	SVC, internal jugular veins
Posterior	Portion of IVC, common iliac veins
Subcardinal	Portion of IVC, renal veins, gonadal veins
Supracardinal	Portion of IVC, intercostal veins, hemiazygos vein, azygos vein

IVC = inferior vena cava; SVC = superior vena cava.

[a]Early in development, the recurrent laryngeal nerves hook around aortic arch 6. On the right side, the distal part of aortic arch 6 regresses, and the right recurrent laryngeal nerve moves up to hook around the right subclavian artery. On the left side, aortic arch 6 persists as the ductus arteriosus (or ligamentum arteriosus in the adult); the left recurrent laryngeal nerve remains hooked around the ductus arteriosus.

[b]Note that the IVC is derived embryologically from four different sources.

Case Study 1

A distraught father comes in with his 10-year-old son, saying that his son began "turning blue" when he was out playing catch with him. His son remarked that he "just felt really tired" when he was running after the ball. He is concerned that his son wouldn't be able to play in the big game this weekend. What is the most likely diagnosis?

Differentials

- Congenital septal defect (ASD, VSD, PDA), Eisenmenger complex, coarctation of the aorta, asthma

Relevant Physical Exam Findings
- Loud holosystolic ejection murmur on auscultation
- Cyanosis
- Clubbing of fingernails

Relevant Lab Findings
- Electrocardiogram shows right ventricular hypertrophy

Diagnosis
- **VSD:** On auscultation, the child had a holosystolic murmur, which can eventually result in an Eisenmenger complex; that is, a shift from a left-to-right shunt to a right-to-left shunt. The symptom of cyanosis became apparent in childhood rather than in infancy. An ASD would have a fixed, split S2, systolic ejection murmur. A PDA that is normally detected in infants would have a continuous machine-like murmur. Coarctation of the aorta would show a holosystolic murmur; however, there was no finding of a lack of a femoral pulse or rib notching.

Case Study 2

Parents bring their 7-day-old infant daughter to the emergency room complaining that their daughter suddenly is breathing so rapidly that it scared them. The mother tells you that her baby previously fed for 10 minutes at each breast every 2 hours, but today she just cries and latches on for only a few seconds. The mother also says, "My baby was very fussy this morning, I don't know what's wrong." What is the most likely diagnosis?

Differentials
- Torsade de pointes, atrial fibrillation, pulmonary obstruction, sinus tachycardia, cystic fibrosis

Relevant Physical Exam Findings
- Heart rate: 305 bpm
- Respiratory rate: 70 breaths/min
- No fever
- No episodes of vomiting
- Urine output normal
- Nonbloody stools
- No prior episodes of difficulty breathing
- Distal extremities are pink with normal capillary refill
- Baby does not appear distressed or uncomfortable
- Oropharynx is clear
- No nasal congestion

Relevant Lab Findings
- EKG shows excessively rapid regular tachycardia with no discernible P waves

Diagnosis
- **Supraventricular tachycardia (SVT):** SVT is defined as a rapid, regular rhythm that requires only atrial or atrioventricular tissue for its initiation. The most common dysrhythmia in children is paroxysmal SVT (PSVT) and is usually caused by an atrioventricular re-entry pathway.

Chapter 7
Digestive System

I Primitive Gut Tube (Figure 7-1)

A. The **primitive gut tube** is formed from the incorporation of the dorsal part of the yolk sac into the embryo due to the craniocaudal folding and lateral folding of the embryo.

B. The primitive gut tube extends from the oropharyngeal membrane to the cloacal membrane and is divided into the **foregut**, **midgut**, and **hindgut**.

C. Early in development, the epithelial lining of the gut tube proliferates rapidly and obliterates the lumen. Later, **recanalization** occurs.

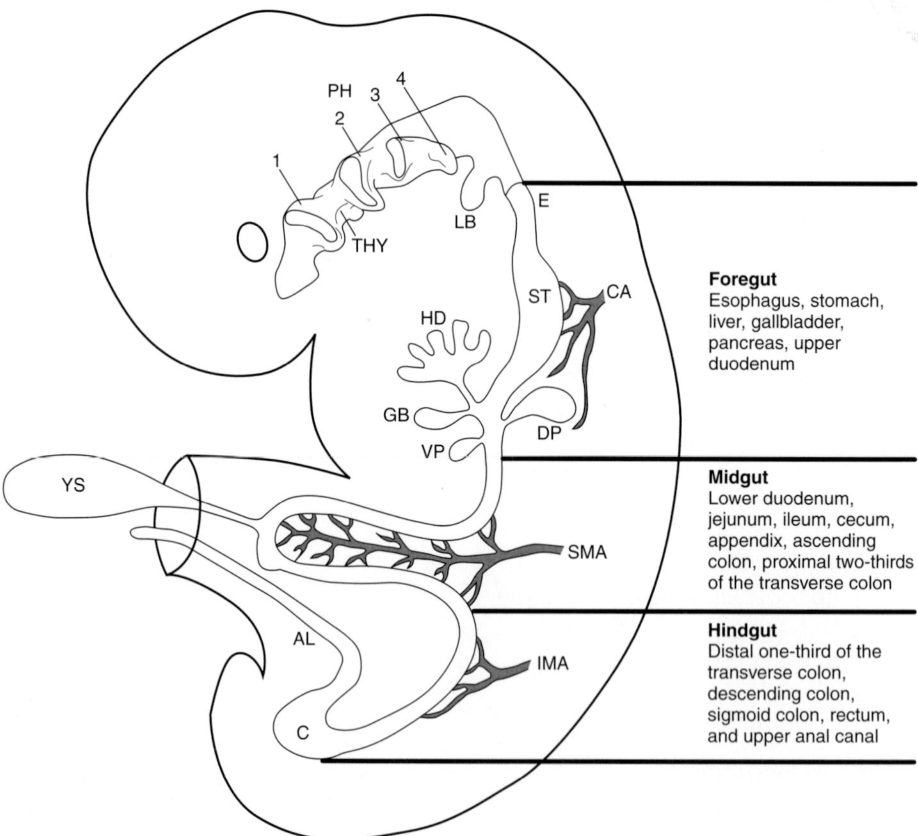

● **Figure 7-1** Development of the gastrointestinal tract, showing the foregut, midgut, and hindgut along with the adult derivatives. The entire length of the endodermal gut tube is shown from the mouth to the anus. THY = thyroid diverticulum; PH = pharyngeal pouches; LB = lung bud; E = esophagus; ST = stomach; CA = celiac artery; HD = hepatic diverticulum; GB = gallbladder; DP = dorsal pancreatic bud; VP = ventral pancreatic bud; SMA = superior mesenteric artery; IMA = inferior mesenteric artery; C = cloaca; AL = allantois; YS = yolk sac.

II Foregut Derivatives

Foregut Derivatives are supplied by the **celiac artery** and include the esophagus, stomach, liver, gall bladder, pancreas, and upper duodenum.

III Esophagus

A. FORMATION. The foregut is divided into the esophagus dorsally and the trachea ventrally by the **tracheoesophageal folds**, which fuse to form the **tracheoesophageal septum.**

B. CLINICAL CONSIDERATIONS

1. **Esophageal atresia** occurs when the tracheoesophageal septum deviates too far dorsally, causing the esophagus to end as a closed tube. About 33% of patients with esophageal atresia also have other congenital defects associated with the VATER (vertebral defects, anal atresia, tracheoesophageal fistula, and renal defects) or VACTERL (similar to VATER but also cardiovascular defects and upper limb defects) syndrome. It is associated clinically with polyhydramnios (fetus is unable to swallow amniotic fluid) and a tracheoesophageal fistula. The photograph in Figure 7-2A (posterior view) shows that the esophagus terminates blindly in a blunted esophageal pouch (arrow). There is a distal esophageal connection with the trachea at the carina (arrowhead).

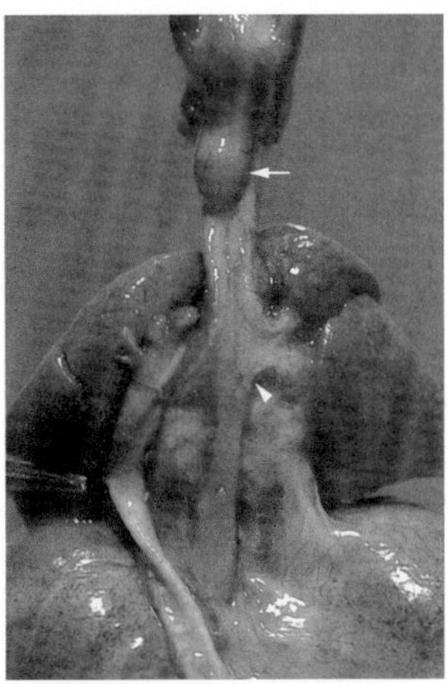

● **Figure 7-2A** Esophageal atresia.

2. **Esophageal stenosis** occurs when the lumen of the esophagus is narrowed and usually involves the midesophagus. The stenosis may be caused by submucosal/muscularis externa hypertrophy, remnants of the tracheal cartilaginous ring within the wall of the esophagus, or a membranous diaphragm obstructing the lumen probably due to incomplete recanalization. The micrograph in Figure 7-2B shows the stratified squamous epithelial lining of the esophagus and submucosal glands. Note that a portion of the muscular wall contains remnants of cartilage (arrow), which contributes to a stenosis.

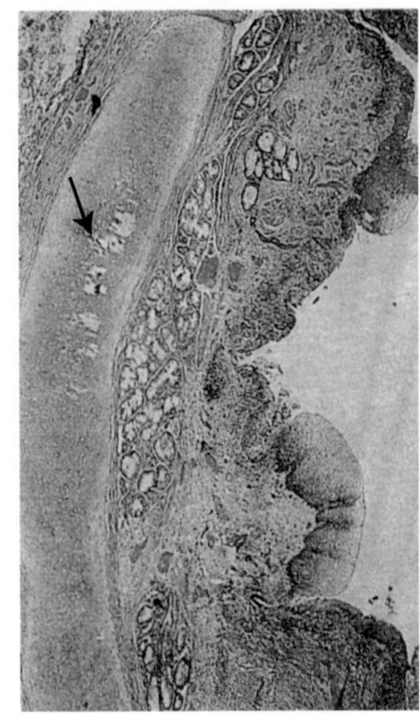

● **Figure 7-2B** Esophageal stenosis.

3. **Achalasia** occurs due to the loss of ganglion cells in the myenteric (Auerbach) plexus and is characterized by the failure to relax the lower esophageal sphincter, which will cause progressive dysphagia and difficulty in swallowing.

IV Stomach

A. FORMATION (FIGURE 7-3A)

1. A fusiform dilatation forms in the foregut in week 4, which gives rise to the **primitive stomach**.
2. The primitive stomach rotates 90° clockwise around its longitudinal axis.
3. As a result of this clockwise rotation, the dorsal mesentery is carried to the left and eventually forms the **greater omentum**; the **left vagus nerve** (CN X) innervates the ventral surface of the stomach; and the **right vagus nerve** (CN X) innervates the dorsal surface of the stomach.

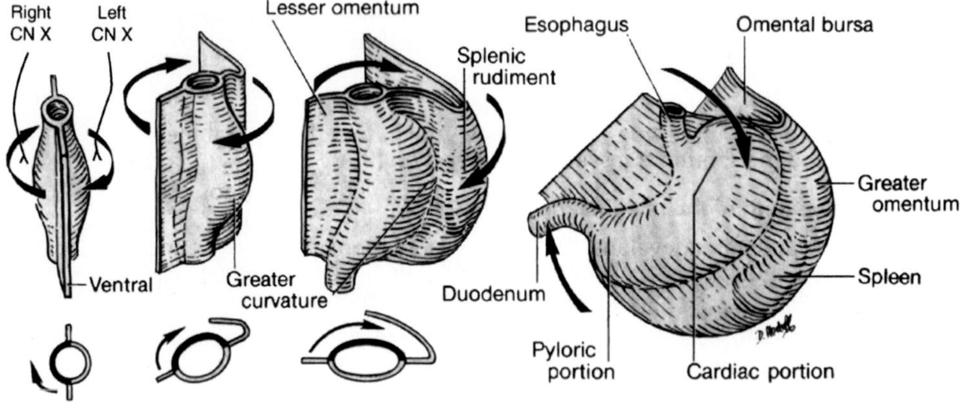

Figure 7-3A Diagram depicting the development and 90° rotation of the stomach from week 4 through week 6. CN X = cranial nerve X (vagus).

B. CLINICAL CONSIDERATION.

Hypertrophic pyloric stenosis occurs when the muscularis externa in the pyloric region hypertrophies, causing a narrow pyloric lumen that obstructs food passage. It is associated clinically with projectile, nonbilious vomiting after feeding and a small, palpable mass at the right costal margin; increased incidence has been found in infants treated with the antibiotic erythromycin. Treatment involves surgical incision of the hypertrophic muscle. The barium contrast radiograph in Figure 7-3B shows the long, narrow channel of the pylorus (arrows) in a patient with hypertrophic pyloric stenosis.

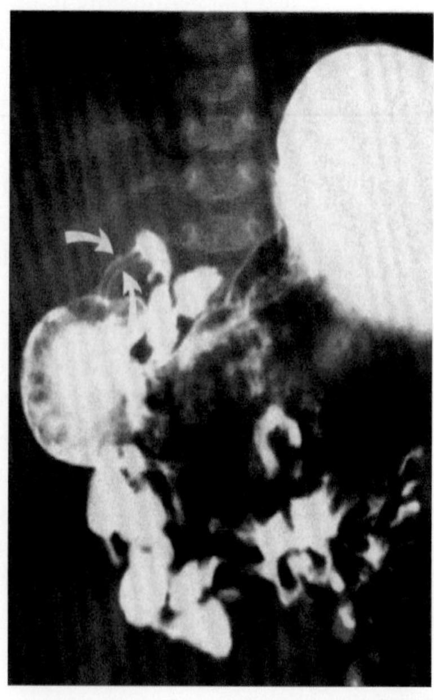

Figure 7-3B Hypertrophic pyloric stenosis.

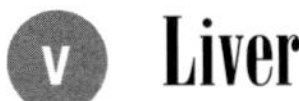

Liver

A. FORMATION (FIGURE 7-4)

1. The endodermal lining of the foregut forms an outgrowth (called the **hepatic diverticulum**) into the surrounding mesoderm of the **septum transversum.**
2. Cords of hepatoblasts (called **hepatic cords**) from the hepatic diverticulum grow into the mesoderm of the septum transversum.
3. The hepatic cords arrange themselves around the **vitelline veins and umbilical veins**, which course through the septum transversum and form the **hepatic sinusoids.**
4. The liver bulges into the abdominal cavity, thereby stretching the septum transversum to form the **ventral mesentery**, consisting of the **falciform ligament** and the **lesser omentum.**
5. The falciform ligament contains the **left umbilical vein**, which regresses after birth to form the **ligamentum teres.**
6. The lesser omentum can be divided into the **hepatogastric ligament** and **hepatoduodenal ligament**. The hepatoduodenal ligament contains the **bile duct, portal vein, and hepatic artery (i.e., portal triad).**

B. CLINICAL CONSIDERATION. Congenital malformations of the liver are rare.

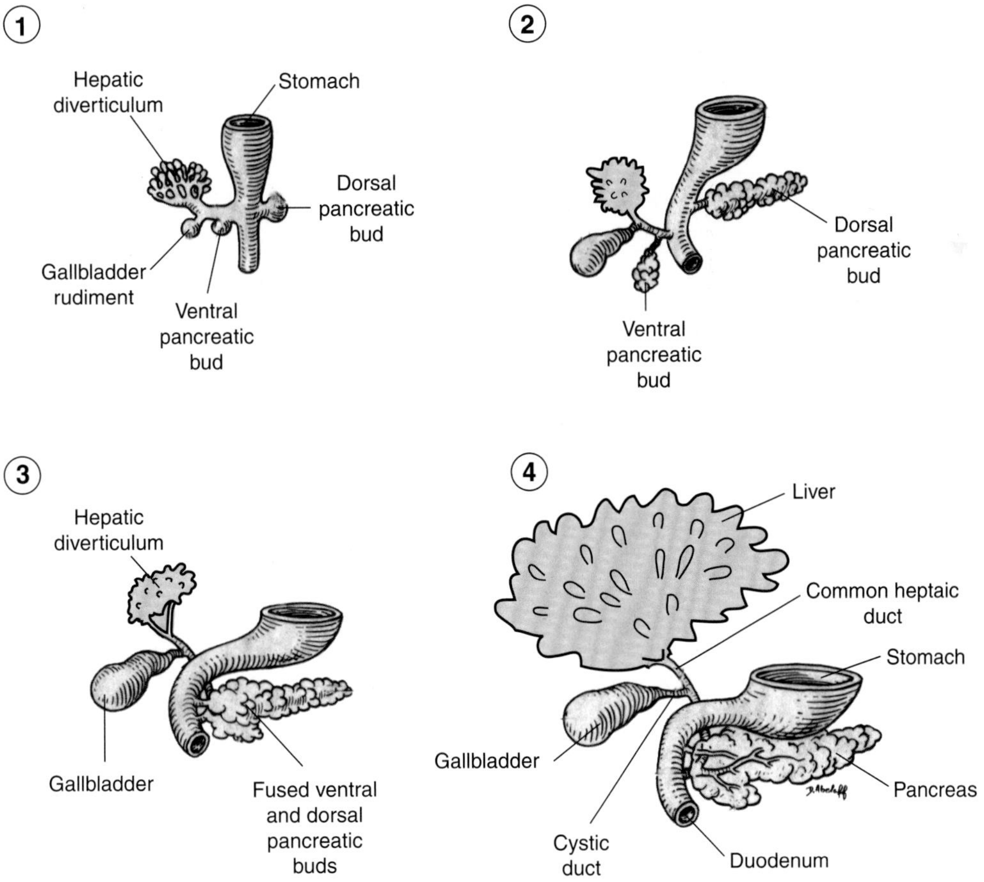

● **Figure 7-4** Sequence of events in the development of the hepatic diverticulum and gall bladder rudiment from week 4 through week 7.

Gall Bladder and Bile Ducts

A. FORMATION (FIGURE 7-4)

1. The connection between the hepatic diverticulum and the foregut narrows to form the bile duct.
2. An outgrowth from the bile duct gives rise to the **gallbladder rudiment** and **cystic duct**.

B. CLINICAL CONSIDERATIONS

1. **Intrahepatic gall bladder** occurs when the gallbladder rudiment advances beyond the hepatic diverticulum and becomes buried within the substance of the liver.
2. **Floating gall bladder** occurs when the gallbladder rudiment lags behind the hepatic diverticulum and thereby becomes suspended from the liver by a mesentery. A floating gall bladder is at risk for **torsion**.
3. **Developmental anomalies of the cystic duct** anatomy are fairly common.
4. **Developmental anomalies of the gall bladder** anatomy are fairly common in which two, bilobed, diverticula, and septated gall bladders are found.
5. **Biliary atresia** is defined as the obliteration of extrahepatic and/or intrahepatic ducts. The ducts are replaced by fibrotic tissue due to acute and chronic inflammation. Clinical findings include: progressive neonatal jaundice with onset soon after birth, white, clay-colored stool, and dark-colored urine; average survival time is 12–19 months with a 100% mortality rate; can be treated by liver transplantation.

Pancreas

A. FORMATION (FIGURE 7-4)

1. The **ventral pancreatic bud** and **dorsal pancreatic bud** are direct outgrowths of foregut endoderm.
2. Within both pancreatic buds, endodermal tubules surrounded by mesoderm branch repeatedly to form acinar cells and ducts (i.e., exocrine pancreas).
3. Isolated clumps of endodermal cells bud from the tubules and accumulate within the mesoderm to form **islet cells** (i.e., endocrine pancreas).
4. Because of the 90° clockwise rotation of the duodenum, the ventral bud rotates dorsally and fuses with the dorsal bud to form the definitive adult pancreas.
5. The ventral bud forms the **uncinate process** and a **portion of the head of the pancreas**.
6. The dorsal bud forms the **remaining portion of the head, body, and tail of the pancreas**.
7. The main pancreatic duct is formed by the anastomosis of the **distal two-thirds of the dorsal pancreatic duct** (the proximal one-third regresses) and the **entire ventral pancreatic duct** (48% incidence).

B. CLINICAL CONSIDERATIONS

1. **Accessory pancreatic duct** develops when the proximal one-third of the dorsal pancreatic duct persists and opens into the duodenum through a minor papillae at a site proximal to the ampulla of Vater (33% incidence). The upper diagram in Figure 7-5A shows the normal pattern of the main pancreatic duct (48% incidence in the population). The lower diagram shows an accessory pancreatic duct (33% incidence in the population). Note that the proximal one-third of the dorsal pancreatic duct persists.

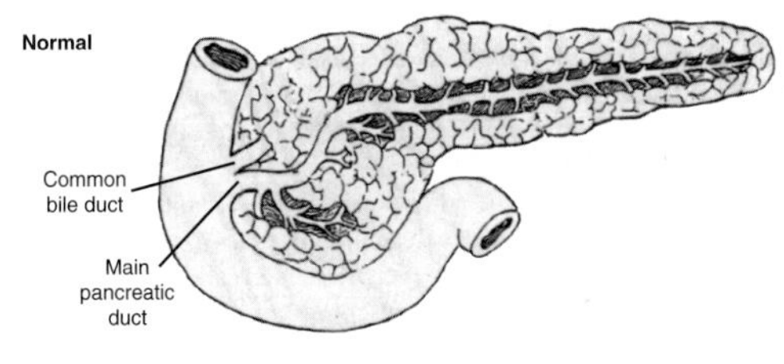

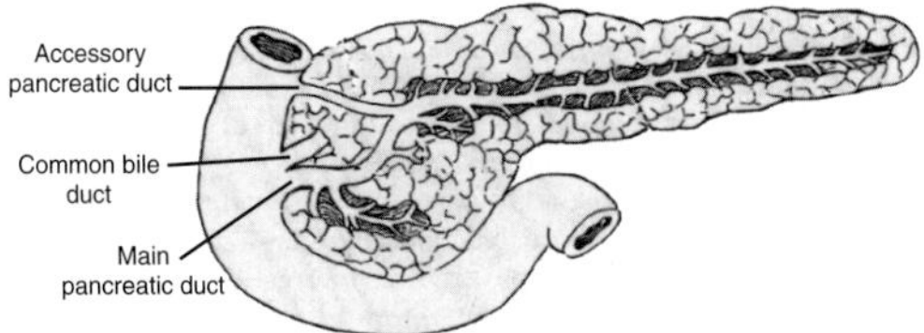

● **Figure 7-5A** Normal and accessory pancreatic duct.

2. **Pancreas divisum** (4% incidence) occurs when the **distal two-thirds of the dorsal pancreatic duct** and the **entire ventral pancreatic duct** fail to anastomose and the proximal one-third of the dorsal pancreatic duct persists, thereby forming two separate duct systems. The dorsal pancreatic duct drains a **portion of the head, body, and tail of the pancreas** by opening into the duodenum through a minor papillae. The ventral pancreatic duct drains the **uncinate process** and a **portion of the head of the pancreas** by opening into the duodenum through the major papillae. Patients with pancreas divisum are prone to pancreatitis, especially if the opening of the dorsal pancreatic duct at the minor papillae is small.

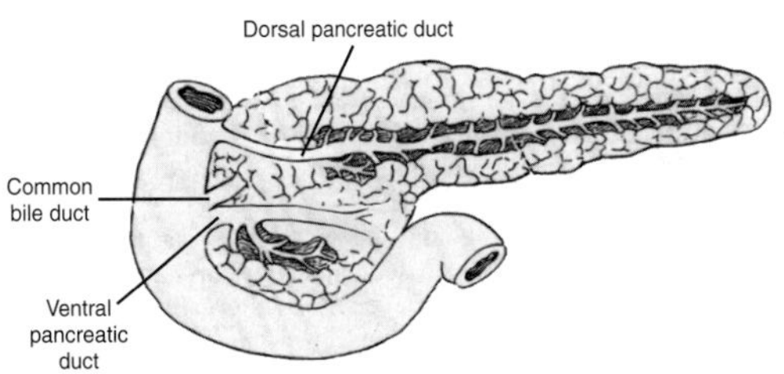

● **Figure 7-5B** Pancreas divisum.

3. **Annular pancreas** occurs when the ventral pancreatic bud fuses with the dorsal bud both dorsally and ventrally, thereby forming a **ring of pancreatic tissue** around the duodenum, causing severe **duodenal obstruction**. Newborns and infants are intolerant of oral feeding and often have bilious vomiting. The radiograph in Figure 7-5C shows that both the stomach (S) and duodenum (D) are distended with air, leading to the "double-bubble" sign, which may be indicative of an annular pancreas.

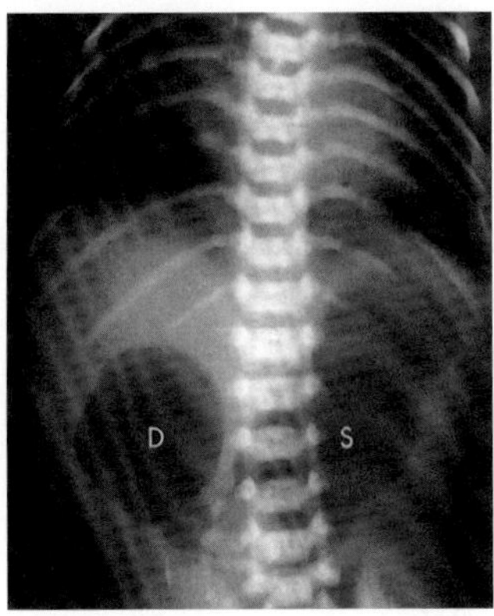

● **Figure 7-5C** Annular pancreas.

VIII Upper Duodenum.

The upper duodenum develops from the caudal portion of the foregut.

IX Midgut Derivatives

are supplied by the **superior mesenteric artery (SMA)** and include the lower duodenum, jejunum, ileum, cecum, appendix, ascending colon, and proximal two-third of the transverse colon.

X Lower Duodenum

A. The **lower duodenum** develops from the cranial-most part of the midgut.

B. The junction of the upper and lower duodenum is just distal to the opening of the common bile duct.

XI Jejunum, Ileum, Cecum, Appendix, Ascending Colon, and Proximal Two-Thirds of Transverse Colon (Figure 7-6)

A. FORMATION

1. The midgut forms a U-shaped loop (**midgut loop**) that herniates through the primitive umbilical ring into the extraembryonic coelom (i.e., **physiological umbilical herniation**) beginning at week 6.
2. The midgut loop consists of a **cranial limb** and a **caudal limb**.
3. The cranial limb forms the **jejunum** and **upper part of the ileum**.

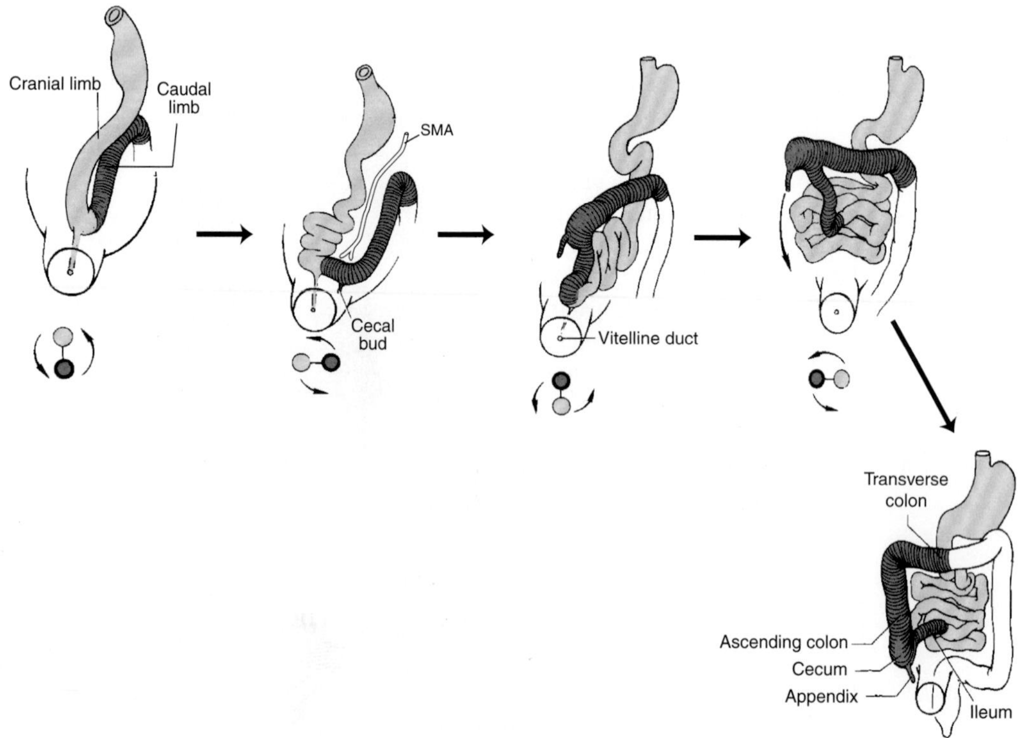

● **Figure 7-6A Diagram depicting the 270° counterclockwise rotation of the midgut loop.** Striped area indicates the caudal limb. Note that after the 270° rotation, the cecum and appendix are located in the upper abdominal cavity. Later in development, there is growth in the direction indicated by the bold arrow so that the cecum and appendix end up in the lower right quadrant. SMA = superior mesenteric artery.

4. The caudal limb forms the **cecal diverticulum**, from which the **cecum** and **appendix** develop; the rest of the caudal limb forms the **lower part of the ileum, ascending colon**, and **proximal 2/3 of the transverse colon**.
5. The midgut loop rotates a total of 270° counterclockwise around the **SMA** as it returns to the abdominal cavity, thus reducing the physiological herniation, around week 11.

B. CLINICAL CONSIDERATIONS

1. **Omphalocele** occurs when abdominal contents herniate through the umbilical ring and persist outside the body covered variably by a translucent peritoneal membrane sac (a light-gray, shiny sac) protruding from the base of the umbilical cord. Large omphaloceles may contain stomach, liver, and intestines. Small omphaloceles contain only intestines. Omphaloceles are usually associated with other congenital anomalies (e.g., trisomy 13, trisomy 18, or Beckwith–Wiedemann syndrome). The photograph in Figure 7-6B shows an omphalocele. Note the clamp on the umbilical cord (UC).
2. **Gastroschisis** occurs when there is a defect in the ventral abdominal wall usually to the right of the umbilical ring through which there is a massive evisceration of intestines (other organs may also be involved). The intestines are not covered by a peritoneal membrane, are directly exposed to amniotic fluid, and are thickened and covered with adhesions.
3. **Ileal diverticulum (Meckel diverticulum)** occurs when a remnant of the vitelline duct persists, thereby forming an outpouching located on the **antimesenteric border** of the ileum. The outpouching may connect to the umbilicus via a fibrous cord or fistula. A Meckel diverticulum is usually located about 30 cm proximal to the ileocecal valve in infants and varies in length from 2 to 15 cm. **Heterotopic gastric mucosa** may be present, which leads to ulceration, perforation, or gastrointestinal bleeding, especially if a large number of parietal cells are present. It is associated clinically with symptoms resembling appendicitis and bright-red or dark-red stools (i.e., bloody). The photograph in Figure 7-6D shows an ileal diverticulum (arrow).

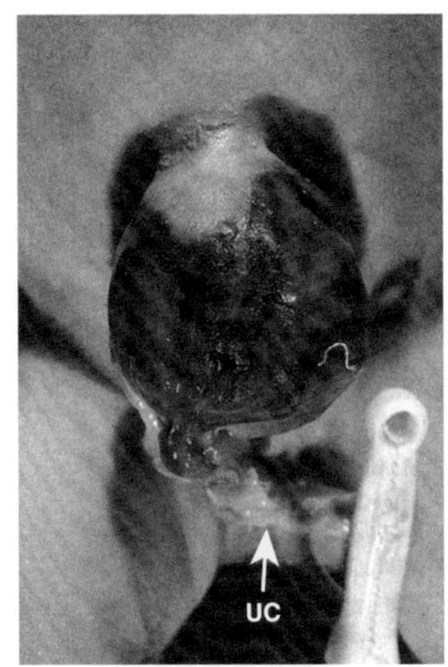

● **Figure 7-6B** Omphalocele.

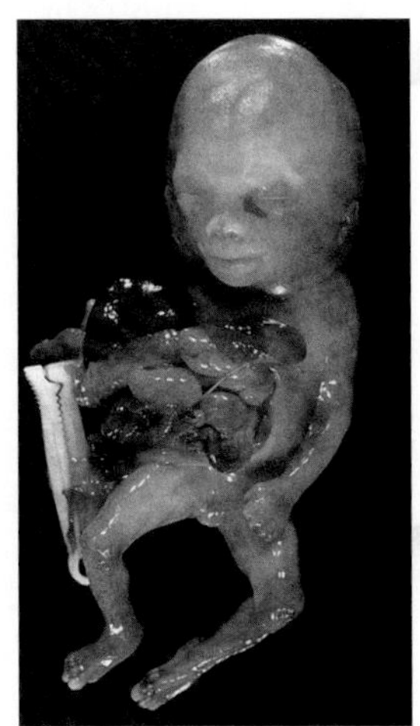

● **Figure 7-6C** Gastroschisis.

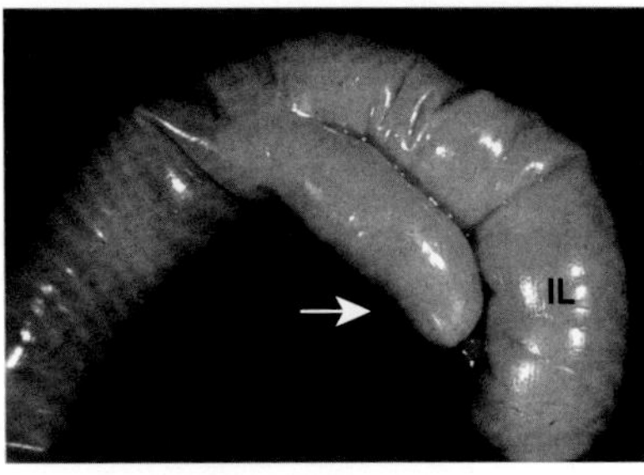

● **Figure 7-6D Ileal diverticulum (Meckel diverticulum).** IL = ileum.

4. **Nonrotation of the midgut loop** occurs when the midgut loop rotates only 90° counterclockwise, thereby positioning the small intestine entirely on the right side and the large intestine entirely on the left side, with the cecum located either in the left upper quadrant or in the left iliac fossa. The radiograph in Figure 7-6E taken after a barium swallow shows the small intestine lying entirely on the right side (arrow).
5. **Malrotation of the midgut loop** occurs when the midgut loop undergoes only partial counterclockwise rotation. This results in the cecum and appendix lying in a subpyloric or subhepatic location and the small intestine suspended by only a vascular pedicle (i.e., not a broad mesentery). A major clinical complication of malrotation is **volvulus** (twisting of the small intestines around the vascular pedicle), which may cause necrosis due to compromised blood supply. (Note: The abnormal position of the appendix due to malrotation of the midgut should be considered when diagnosing appendicitis.) When malrotation is surgically corrected, the appendix is removed to prevent delayed or missed diagnosis of appendicitis given the atypical abdominal pain location at presentation. The radiograph in Figure 7-6F taken after a barium swallow shows the typical "beak sign" (arrow; B) that occurs secondary to the twisting of the intestines (volvulus) and an early spiraling of the small intestine (arrowheads).
6. **Reversed rotation of the midgut loop** occurs when the midgut loop rotates clockwise instead of counterclockwise, causing the large intestine to enter the abdominal cavity first. This results in the large intestine being anatomically located posterior to the duodenum and SMA.
7. **Intestinal atresia and stenosis.** Atresia occurs when the lumen of the intestines is completely occluded, whereas stenosis occurs when the lumen of the intestines is narrowed. The causes of

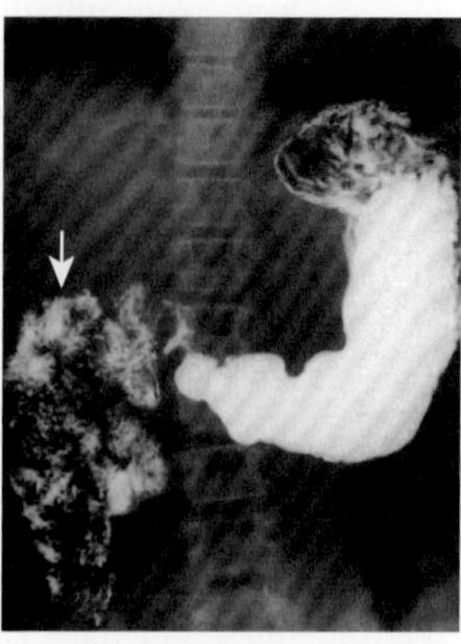

● **Figure 7-6E** Nonrotation of the midgut loop.

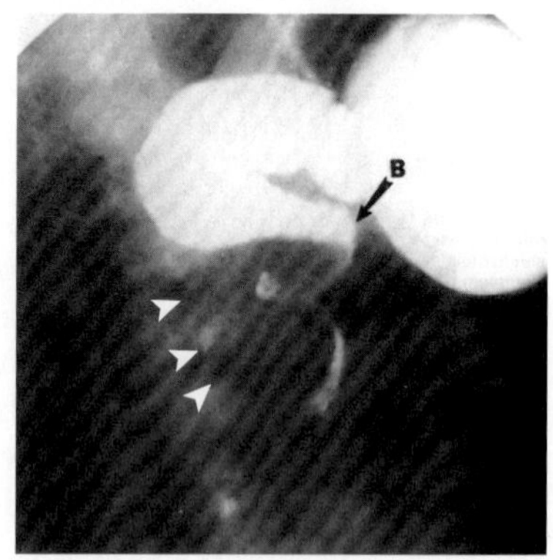

● **Figure 7-6F** Malrotation of the midgut loop (volvulus).

these conditions seem to be both failed recanalization and/or an ischemic intrauterine event ("vascular accident"). Clinical findings of proximal atresias include: polyhydramnios and bilious vomiting early after birth. Clinical findings of distal atresias include normal amniotic fluid levels, abdominal distention, later vomiting, and failure to pass meconium.

8. **Duplication of the intestines** occurs when a segment of the intestines is duplicated as a result of abnormal recanalization (most commonly near the ileocecal valve). The duplication is found on the mesenteric border; its lumen generally communicates with the normal bowel, shares the same blood supply as the normal bowel, and is lined by normal intestinal epithelium, but heterotopic gastric and pancreatic tissue has been identified. Clinical findings include: an abdominal mass, bouts of abdominal pain, vomiting, chronic rectal bleeding, intussusception, and perforation.
9. **Intussusception** occurs when a segment of bowel invaginates or telescopes into an adjacent bowel segment, leading to obstruction or ischemia. This is one of the most common causes of obstruction in children younger than 2 years of age, is most often idiopathic, and most commonly involves the ileum and colon (i.e., ileocolic). Clinical findings include: acute onset of intermittent abdominal pain, vomiting, bloody stools, diarrhea, and somnolence.
10. **Retrocecal and retrocolic appendix** occurs when the appendix is located on the posterior side of the cecum or colon, respectively. These anomalies are very common and important to remember during appendectomies. Note: The appendix is normally found on the medial side of the cecum.
11. **SMA syndrome** occurs when the third portion of the duodenum is compressed due to a decreased angle (as low as 6°) between the SMA and the aorta. This syndrome is caused by a loss of the intervening mesenteric fat pad due to a significant weight loss (e.g., bariatric surgery, anorexia nervosa), severe debilitating illnesses (e.g., malignant cancer), spinal cord injury, or corrective surgery for scoliosis.

XII Hindgut Derivatives

Hindgut Derivatives are supplied by the **inferior mesenteric artery** and include the distal 1/3 of the transverse colon, descending colon, sigmoid colon, rectum, and upper anal canal.

XIII Distal One-third of Transverse Colon, Descending Colon, Sigmoid Colon

A. The cranial end of the hindgut develops into the distal 1/3 of the transverse colon, descending colon, and sigmoid colon.

B. The terminal end of the hindgut is an endoderm-lined pouch called the **cloaca**, which contacts the surface ectoderm of the **proctodeum** to form the **cloacal membrane**.

XIV Rectum and Upper Anal Canal

A. FORMATION (FIGURE 7-7A)

1. The cloaca is partitioned by the **urorectal septum** into the **rectum and upper anal canal** and the **urogenital sinus**.
2. The cloacal membrane is partitioned by the urorectal septum into **anal membrane** and **urogenital membrane**.
3. The urorectal septum fuses with the cloacal membrane at the future site of the gross anatomic **perineal body**.

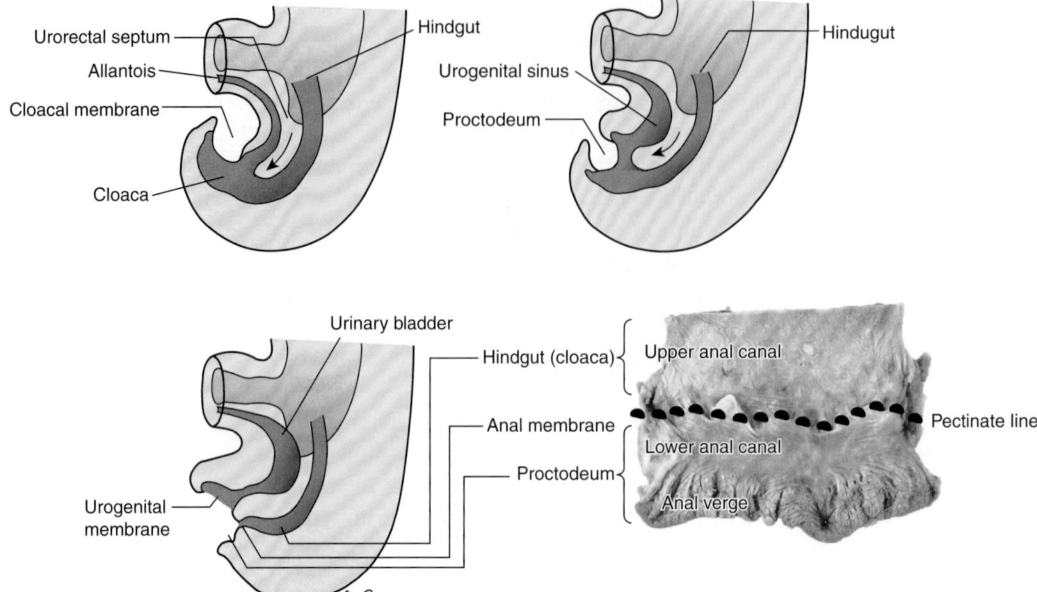

● **Figure 7-7A Diagram depicting the partitioning of the cloaca by the urorectal septum.** The bold arrow shows the direction of growth of the urorectal septum.

B. CLINICAL CONSIDERATIONS

1. **Colonic aganglionosis (Hirschsprung disease)** is caused by the arrest of the caudal migration of neural crest cells. The hallmark is the absence of ganglionic cells in the myenteric and submucosal plexuses most commonly in the sigmoid colon and rectum, resulting in a narrow segment of colon (i.e., the colon fails to relax). Although the ganglionic cells are absent, there is a proliferation of hypertrophied nerve fiber bundles. The most characteristic functional finding is the failure of internal anal sphincter to relax following rectal distension (i.e., abnormal rectoanal reflex). Clinical findings include: a distended abdomen, inability to pass meconium, gushing of fecal material upon a rectal digital exam, and a loss of peristalsis in the colon segment distal to the normal innervated colon. Figure 7-7B shows the radiograph after barium enema of a patient with Hirschsprung disease. The upper segment of the normal colon (*) is distended with fecal material. The lower segment of the colon (**) is narrow. The lower segment is the portion of the colon where the

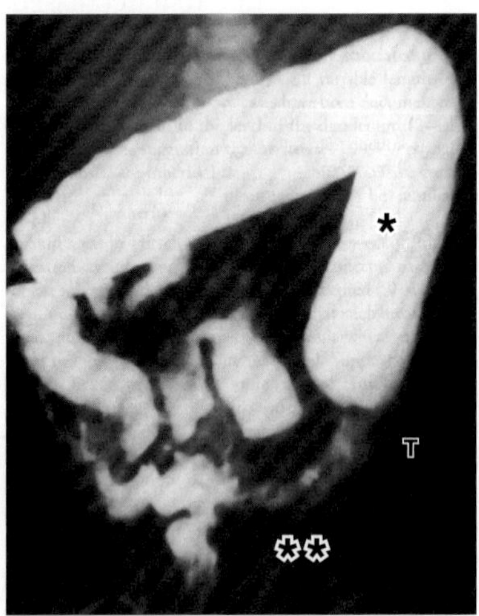

● **Figure 7-7B** Hirschsprung disease.

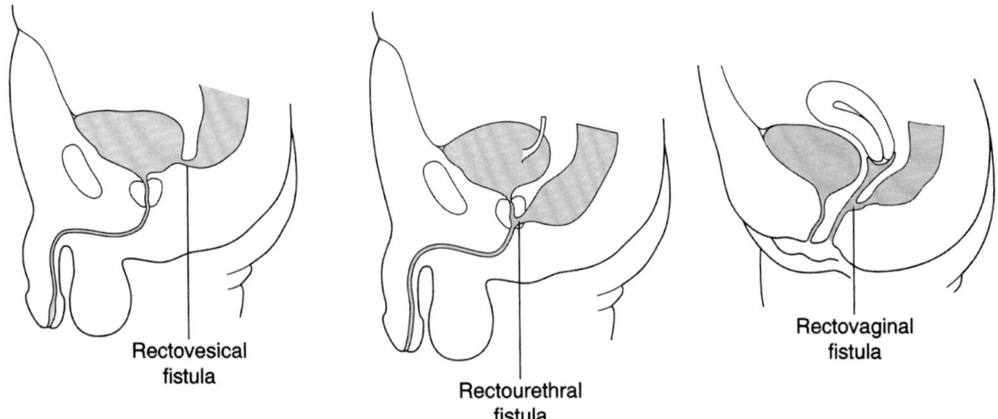

● **Figure 7-7C** Rectovesical fistula, rectourethral fistula, and rectovaginal fistula.

ganglionic cells in the myenteric and submucosal plexuses are absent. This case shows a low transition zone (T) between the normal colon and aganglionic colon.

2. **Rectovesical, rectourethral, and rectovaginal fistulas** (Figure 7-7C) are, respectively, abnormal communications between the rectum and urinary bladder (rectovesical), rectum and urethra (rectourethral), and rectum and vagina (rectovaginal) due to abnormal formation of the urorectal septum. These fistulas are associated clinically with the presence of meconium in the urine or vagina. A rectourethral fistula that generally occurs in males is associated with the prostatic urethra and is therefore sometimes called a **rectoprostatic fistula.**

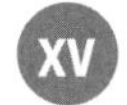

XV The Anal Canal

A. FORMATION (SEE FIGURE 7-7A)

1. The **upper anal canal** develops from the **hindgut.**
2. The **lower anal canal** develops from the **proctodeum**, which is an invagination of surface ectoderm caused by a proliferation of mesoderm surrounding the anal membrane.
3. The junction between the upper and lower anal canals is indicated by the **pectinate line**, which also marks the site of the former **anal membrane.**
4. In the adult, the pectinate line is located at the lower border of the anal columns.

B. CLINICAL CONSIDERATIONS

1. **Imperforate anus** occurs when the anal membrane fails to perforate; a layer of tissue separates the anal canal from the exterior.
2. **Anal agenesis** occurs when the anal canal ends as a blind sac **below the puborectalis muscle** due to abnormal formation of the urorectal septum. It is usually associated with rectovesical, rectourethral, or rectovaginal fistula.
3. **Anorectal agenesis** occurs when the rectum ends as a blind sac **above the puborectalis muscle** due to abnormal formation of the urorectal septum. It is the most common type of anorectal malformation and is usually associated with a rectovesical, rectourethral, or rectovaginal fistula.
4. **Rectal atresia** occurs when both the rectum and anal canal are present but remain unconnected due to either abnormal recanalization or a compromised blood supply causing focal atresia.

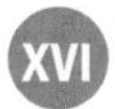

Mesenteries. The primitive gut tube is suspended within the peritoneal cavity of the embryo by a **ventral** and **dorsal mesentery** from which all adult mesenteries are derived (Table 7-1).

TABLE 7-1 DERIVATION OF ADULT MESENTERIES

Embryonic Mesentery	Adult Mesentery
Ventral mesentery	Lesser omentum (hepatoduodenal and hepatogastric ligaments), falciform ligament, coronary ligament of the liver, and triangular ligaments of the liver
Dorsal mesentery	Greater omentum (gastrorenal, gastrosplenic, gastrocolic, and splenorenal ligaments), mesentery of small intestine, mesoappendix, transverse mesocolon, sigmoid mesocolon

Case Study 1

A 39-year-old man comes to your office complaining of "heartburn after trying to eat" and not being able to swallow anything. He states, "I have tried everything from water to steaks, it doesn't matter what I eat I always have trouble swallowing it down." What is the most likely diagnosis?

Differentials

- Neurological disorder, thyroid disease, thyroid mass, infection, reflux esophagitis

Relevant Physical Exam Findings

- Dysphagia
- Normal thyroid on palpation

Relevant Lab Findings

- Barium swallow X-ray shows a dilated esophagus with an area of distal stenosis. Almost looks like a "bird's beak."
- Normal thyroid levels

Diagnosis

- **Achalasia:** The findings on the X-ray are a telltale sign of achalasia. Another telltale sign is that patients have dysphagia involving both solids and liquids. The physical and lab findings excluded thyroid disease and masses. Even though reflux esophagitis would present with heartburn, it is only limited to dysphagia of solids, not solids and liquid.

Case Study 2

A mother brings her 1-month-old son into the clinic, complaining of him "vomiting all over the place when he tries to eat something." She says her son's vomiting looks like it was "shot out of a cannon." What is the most likely diagnosis?

Differentials

- Hiatal hernia, malrotation with volvulus

Relevant Physical Exam Findings

- Small, nontender palpable mass on right costal margin

Relevant Lab Findings

- Barium swallow X-ray shows a narrow pyloric channel.
- Abdominal ultrasound shows a hypertrophic pylorus.

Diagnosis

- Hypertrophic pyloric stenosis

Case Study 3

A man brings his 3-year-old son into the office, complaining of his son having "bad stomach pains" and talks about him "running a fever" and being "thirsty all the time." He remarks that his son has not had a bowel movement lately. What is the most likely diagnosis?

Differentials

- Volvulus, intussusception, indirect hernia, foreign-body obstruction

Relevant Physical Exam Findings

- Painless rectal bleeding
- Abdominal distension

Relevant Lab Findings

- X-ray findings showed remnant of vitelline duct that was estimated to be about 2 feet from the ileocecal valve.
- No detection of patent processus vaginalis
- Biopsy shows ectopic gastric and pancreatic mucosal tissue.

Diagnosis

- **Meckel diverticulum:** A Meckel diverticulum occurs when a remnant of embryonic vitelline duct persists. This condition is associated with volvulus and intussusception. However, due to the finding of the remnants, those two conditions can be excluded. There was no detection of a foreign body being found in the gastrointestinal tract on X-ray. Also, an indirect hernia was ruled out because of the nondetection of a patent process vaginalis, which is needed to make a diagnosis of an indirect hernia.

Case Study 4

A nurse comes into your office informing you that the child you delivered yesterday failed to pass meconium. The nurse remarks that the child also cries on palpation of the abdominal area. What is the most likely diagnosis?

Differentials
- Anal atresia, anal malformation, anal stenosis, cystic fibrosis

Relevant Physical Exam Findings
- Abdominal distension
- Bilious vomiting
- Megacolon on palpation

Relevant Lab Findings
- Barium enema shows dilated proximal segment and a narrow distal segment.

Diagnosis
- Hirschsprung disease

Chapter 8

Urinary System

I Overview (Figure 8-1)

A. The **intermediate mesoderm** forms a longitudinal elevation along the dorsal body wall called the **urogenital ridge**.

B. A portion of the urogenital ridge forms the **nephrogenic cord**, which gives rise to the urinary system.

C. The nephrogenic cord develops into three sets of nephric structures: the **pronephros, the mesonephros**, and **the metanephros.**

II The Pronephros

A. Develops by the differentiation of mesoderm within the nephrogenic cord to form **pronephric tubules** and the **pronephric duct.**

B. The pronephros is the cranial-most nephric structure and is a transitory structure that regresses completely by week 5.

C. The pronephros is not functional in humans.

III The Mesonephros

A. Develops by the differentiation of mesoderm within the nephrogenic cord to form **mesonephric tubules** and the **mesonephric duct (Wolffian duct).**

B. The mesonephros is the middle nephric structure and is a partially transitory structure. Most of the mesonephric tubules regress, but the mesonephric duct persists and opens into the urogenital sinus.

C. The mesonephros is functional for a short period.

IV The Metanephros

A. Develops from an outgrowth of the mesonephric duct (called the **ureteric bud**) and from a condensation of mesoderm within the nephrogenic cord called the **metanephric mesoderm.**

B. The metanephros is the caudal-most nephric structure.

C. The metanephros begins to form at week 5 and is functional in the fetus at about week 10. The metanephros develops into the **definitive adult kidney**.

D. The fetal kidney is divided into lobes, in contrast to the definitive adult kidney, which has a smooth contour.

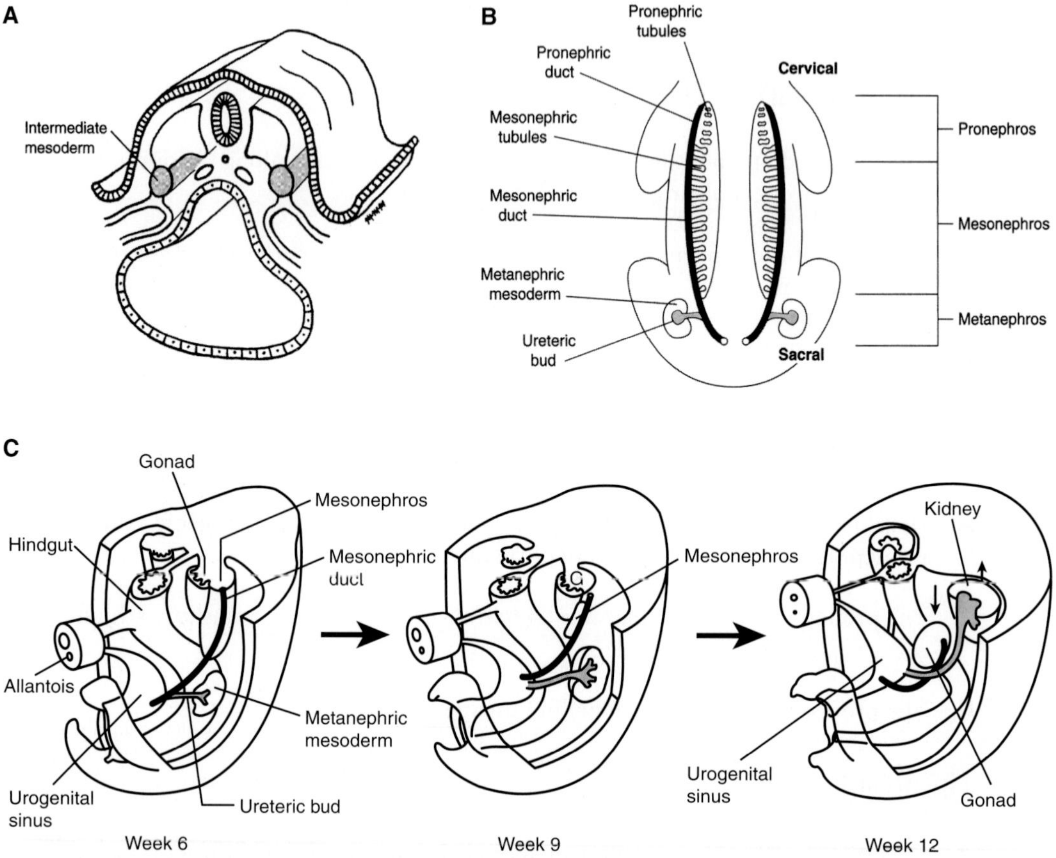

● **Figure 8-1 Early development of the kidney. (A)** Cross-sectional view of an embryo at week 4, illustrating the intermediate mesoderm as a cord of mesoderm that extends from the cervical to the sacral levels and forms the urogenital ridge and nephrogenic cord. **(B)** Frontal view of an embryo, depicting the pronephros, the mesonephros, and the metanephros. Note that nephric structures develop from cervical through sacral levels. **(C)** Diagrams showing the relationship between the gonad, the mesonephros, and the metanephros during development at weeks 6, 9, and 12. Note that the gonad descends (*arrow*), while the metanephros ascends (*arrow*).

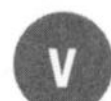

Development of the Metanephros (Figure 8-2)

A. DEVELOPMENT OF THE COLLECTING SYSTEM

1. The ureteric bud is an outgrowth of the mesonephric duct.
2. The ureteric bud initially penetrates the metanephric mesoderm and then undergoes repeated branching to form the **ureters**, **renal pelvis**, **major calyces**, **minor calyces**, and **collecting ducts**.

B. DEVELOPMENT OF THE NEPHRON

1. The inductive influence of the collecting ducts causes the metanephric mesoderm to differentiate into **metanephric vesicles**, which later give rise to primitive **S-shaped renal tubules** that are critical to nephron formation.
2. The S-shaped renal tubules differentiate into the **connecting tubule, the distal convoluted tubule, the loop of Henle, the proximal convoluted tubule**, and the **Bowman's capsule.** Tufts of capillaries called **glomeruli** protrude into Bowman's capsule.
3. Nephron formation is complete at birth, but functional maturation of nephrons continues throughout infancy.

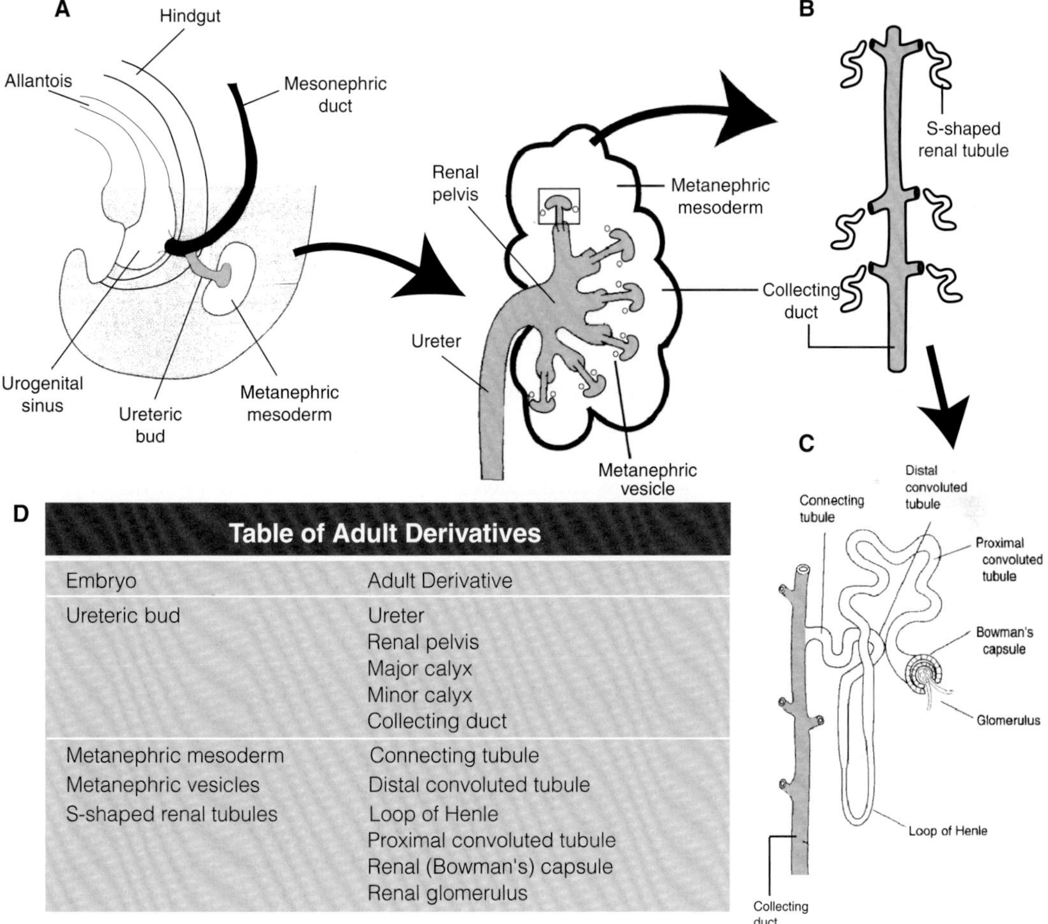

Table of Adult Derivatives

Embryo	Adult Derivative
Ureteric bud	Ureter Renal pelvis Major calyx Minor calyx Collecting duct
Metanephric mesoderm Metanephric vesicles S-shaped renal tubules	Connecting tubule Distal convoluted tubule Loop of Henle Proximal convoluted tubule Renal (Bowman's) capsule Renal glomerulus

● **Figure 8-2 Later development of the kidney. (A)** Lateral view of the embryo showing the relationship between the ureteric bud (*shaded*), the metanephric mesoderm, and the mesonephric duct (*black*). In addition, note the urogenital sinus, hindgut, and allantois. Lateral view of a fetal kidney. Shaded area indicates structures formed from the ureteric bud. **(B)** Note the repeated branching of the ureteric bud into the metanephric mesoderm. At the tip of each collecting duct, the formation of metanephric vesicles is induced. Note the lobulated appearance of a fetal kidney. **(C)** Enlarged view of the rectangle shown in (B), illustrating the further branching of a collecting duct (shaded) and the formation of primitive S-shaped renal tubules. **(D)** Diagram showing a collecting duct and the components of a mature adult nephron. A summary table of derivatives is shown.

VI Relative Ascent of the Kidneys

A. The fetal metanephros is located at vertebral levels **S1-S2**, whereas the definitive adult kidney is located at vertebral level **T12-L3**.

B. The change in location results from a disproportionate growth of the embryo caudal to the metanephros.

C. During the relative ascent, the kidneys **rotate 90°**, causing the hilum, which initially faces ventrally, to finally face medially.

VII Blood Supply of the Kidneys

A. During the relative ascent of the kidneys, the kidneys will receive their blood supply from arteries at progressively higher levels until the definitive renal arteries develop at **L2**.

B. Arteries formed during the ascent may persist and are called **supernumerary arteries.** Supernumerary arteries are **end arteries.** Therefore, any damage to them will result in necrosis of kidney parenchyma.

VIII Development of the Urinary Bladder

A. The urinary bladder is formed from the upper portion of the **urogenital sinus**, which is continuous with the **allantois.**

B. The allantois becomes a fibrous cord called the **urachus** (or **median umbilical ligament** in the adult).

C. The lower ends of the mesonephric ducts become incorporated into the posterior wall of the bladder to form the **trigone of the bladder.**

IX Clinical Considerations (Figures 8-3 to 8-8)

A. RENAL AGENESIS occurs when the ureteric bud fails to develop, thereby eliminating the induction of metanephric vesicles and nephron formation.

1. **Unilateral renal agenesis** is relatively common (more common in males). Therefore, a physician should never assume that a patient has two kidneys. It is asymptomatic and compatible with life because the remaining kidney hypertrophies.
2. **Bilateral renal agenesis** is relatively uncommon. It causes oligohydramnios, which causes compression of the fetus, resulting in **Potter syndrome** (deformed limbs, wrinkly skin, and abnormal facial appearance). These infants are usually stillborn or die shortly after birth.

B. RENAL ECTOPIA occurs when one or both kidneys fail to ascend and therefore remain in the pelvis or lower lumbar area (i.e., **pelvic kidney**). In some cases, two pelvic kidneys fuse to form a solid mass, commonly called a **pancake kidney.**

C. RENAL FUSION. The most common type of renal fusion is the **horseshoe kidney.** A horseshoe kidney occurs when the inferior poles of the kidneys fuse across the midline. Normal ascent of the kidneys is arrested because the fused portion gets trapped below the origin of the **inferior mesenteric artery** from the abdominal aorta. Kidney rotation is also arrested so that the hilum faces ventrally. A horseshoe kidney may also cause urinary tract obstruction due to impingement on the ureters, which may lead to recurrent urinary tract infections as well as pyelonephritis. The computed tomography in Figure 8-3 shows the isthmus of renal tissue (arrow) that extends across the midline.

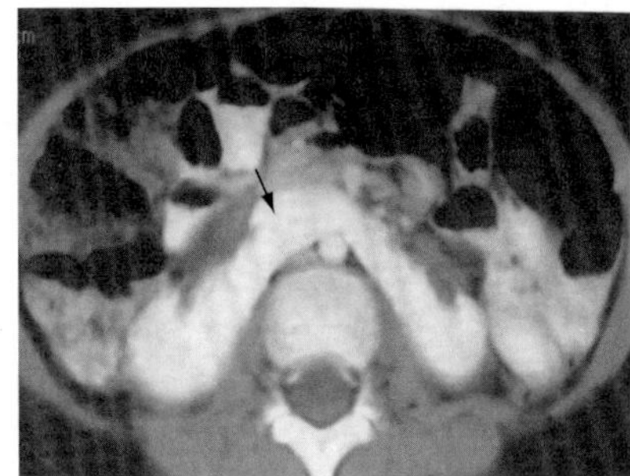

● **Figure 8-3 Horseshoe kidney.**

D. RENAL ARTERY STENOSIS is the most common cause of renovascular hypertension in children. The stenosis may occur in the main renal artery of segmental renal arteries. The angiogram in Figure 8-4 shows bilateral renal artery stenosis (*arrows*).

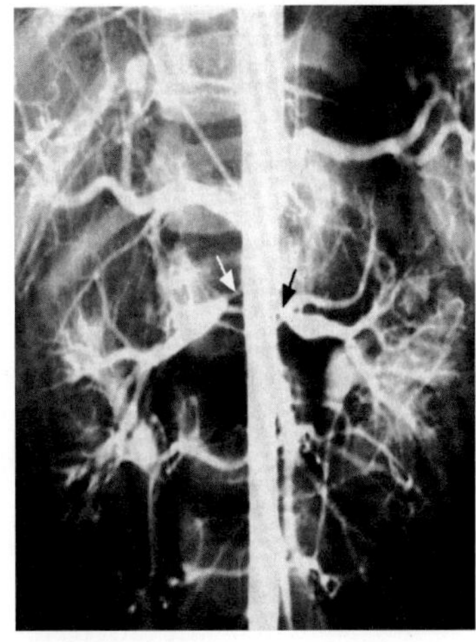

● **Figure 8-4 Renal artery stenosis.**

E. URETEROPELVIC JUNCTION OBSTRUCTION (UPJ) occurs when there is an obstruction to the urine flow from the renal pelvis to the proximal ureter. UPJ is the most common congenital obstruction of the urinary tract. If there is severe uteropelvic atresia, a **multicystic dysplastic kidney** is found, in which the cysts are actually dilated calyces. In this case, the kidney consists of grape-like, smooth-walled cysts of variable size. Between the cysts are found dysplastic glomeruli and atrophic tubules. The photograph in Figure 8-5 shows numerous cysts.

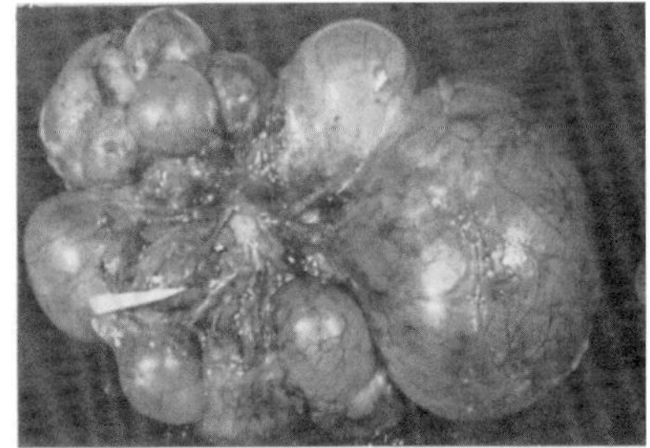

● **Figure 8-5 Multidysplastic kidney.**

F. AUTOSOMAL RECESSIVE POLYCYSTIC KIDNEY DISEASE (ARPKD; formerly called infantile polycystic kidney disease) is an autosomal recessive disease that has been mapped to the short arm of chromosome 6 (p6). In ARPKD, the kidneys (always bilateral) are huge and spongy with a smooth external surface and contain numerous cysts due to the dilatation of collecting ducts and tubules that severely compromise kidney function. ARPKD is associated clinically with cysts of the liver, pancreas, and lungs and hepatic fibrosis (hepatic hypertension). Treatment includes dialysis and kidney transplant. The photograph in Figure 8-6 shows numerous cysts usually confined to the collecting ducts and tubules. Between the cysts, some functioning nephrons can be observed.

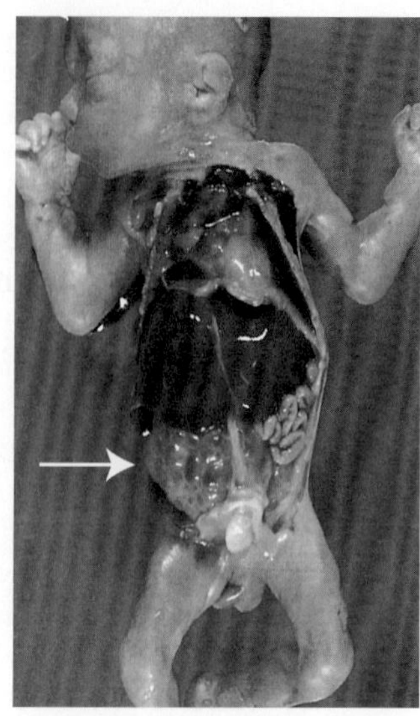

● **Figure 8-6 Autosomal recessive polycystic kidney disease (ARPKD).** Formerly called infantile polycystic kidney disease.

G. WILMS TUMOR (WT). WT is **the most common renal malignancy of childhood.** WT is the most common primary tumor of childhood and is typically due to a deletion of **tumor suppressor gene WT1** located on chromosome 11. WT presents as a large, solitary, well-circumscribed mass that on cut section is soft, homogeneous, and tan-gray in color. WT is interesting histologically, in that this tumor tends to recapitulate different stages of embryological formation of the kidney, so that three classic histological areas are described: a stromal area; a blastemal area of tightly packed embryonic cells; and a tubular area. WT is associated with other congenital anomalies called the WAGR complex (Wilms tumor, aniridia [absence of the iris], genitourinary malformations, and mental retardation). The photograph in Figure 8-7 shows the Wilms tumor extending from normal kidney tissue (arrow).

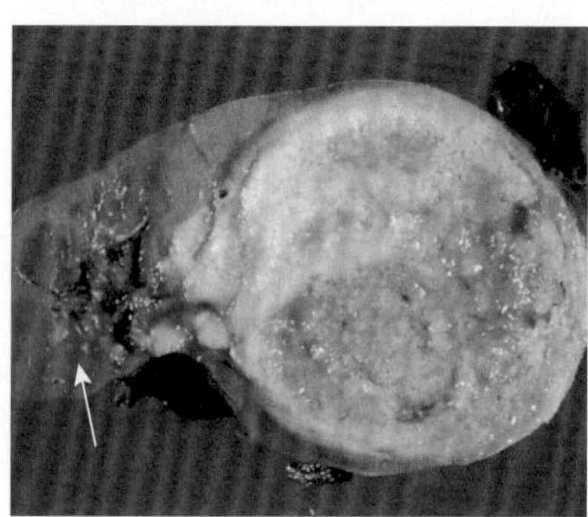

● **Figure 8-7 Wilms tumor.**

H. URETEROPELVIC DUPLICATIONS occur when the ureteric bud prematurely divides before penetrating the metanephric blastema. This results in either a double kidney or a duplicated ureter and renal pelvis. The term *duplex kidney* refers to a configuration where two ureters drain one kidney. The intravenous urogram (IVU) in Figure 8-8 shows duplication of the collecting system on the right side. The two ureters fuse at vertebral level L4 (arrow). However, they may remain separate throughout their course and open separately. The ureter from the lower pole opens normally at the urinary bladder trigone. However, the ureter from the upper pole usually has an ectopic opening.

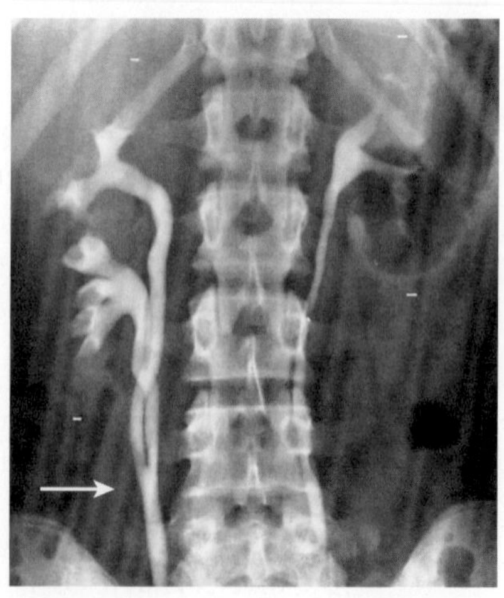

● **Figure 8-8 Ureteropelvic duplication.**

I. URACHAL FISTULA OR CYST occurs when a remnant of the allantois persists, thereby forming fistula or cyst. It is found along the midline on a path from the umbilicus to the apex of the urinary bladder. A urachal fistula forms a direct connection between the urinary bladder and the outside of the body at the umbilicus, causing **urine drainage** from the umbilicus.

J. NUTCRACKER SYNDROME occurs when the left renal vein is compressed between the superior mesenteric artery and the abdominal aorta. Clinical findings include: hematuria leading to anemia, left testicular pain in men, left lower quadrant pain in women, and varicocele.

Case Study 1

A 33-year-old man comes in complaining of "fever and chills" and that he "has to constantly go to the bathroom." He also indicates that he has pain just below the abdominal area on the right side. He states that he has not had sex in more than 6 months. He suspects that it may be urinary tract infection because he "has had a lot of them over the years." What is the most likely diagnosis?

Differentials
- Urinary tract infection (UTI), pyelonephritis, kidney stones

Relevant Physical Exam Findings
- Flank pain
- Costovertebral angle (CVA) tenderness

Relevant Lab Findings
- Normal calcium levels
- Presence of leukocytes
- Computed tomography scan shows the presence of horseshoe kidney

Diagnosis
- **Horseshoe kidney:** The symptoms that the man had (fevers, chills, flank pain, and CVA tenderness) are classic signs of pyelonephritis as a result of UTI. In this case, the UTI is a result of a urinary tract obstruction caused by a horseshoe kidney.

Case Study 2

A parent brings his 4-year-old daughter into the clinic. He says he has noticed "a lump on his daughter's lower right side that has gotten bigger over time." What is the most likely diagnosis?

Differentials
- Unilateral renal agenesis, neuroblastoma, Wilms tumor

Relevant Physical Exam Findings
- Large palpable mass on the right flank
- Kidney size normal

Relevant Lab Findings
- No presence of UTI
- No increase in catecholamine
- No increase in androgen production
- Genetic testing revealed deletion of tumor suppression gene on chromosome 11

Diagnosis

- **Wilms tumor:** The Wilms tumor is the most common primary renal tumor in childhood and normally presents as a large, palpable, flank mass with hemihypertrophy of the kidney. Unilateral renal agenesis is ruled out because whereas the patient would have renal hypertrophy on one side, the patient would also have only one kidney. Neuroblastoma is ruled out because there was no mention of an increase in urine vanillylmandelic acid and metanephrine levels.

Case Study 3

The parents bring their 9-year-old boy into your office complaining that their son has had intermittent bouts of fever over the last 2 years. Sometimes the fever subsides on its own, but many times they have to get a prescription for an antipyretic or an antibiotic. The father tells you that his son seems smaller than other boys his age and that he gets tired very easily when they play in the yard together. The mother tells you that she is frustrated that no physician can tell her why her son is getting all these fevers and she is concerned there is something more serious going on. She says, "Doc, all these fevers is just not right. Can you help us?" What is the most likely diagnosis?

Differentials

- Megacalycosis (a congenital nonobstructive dilation of the calyces without pelvic or ureteric dilation, vesicoureteral reflux (with marked dilation and kinking of the ureter), midureteral or distal ureteral obstruction (when ureter is not well visualized on the urogram)

Relevant Physical Exam Findings

- Boy is well-nourished
- Slight pallor and Grade 1 digital clubbing
- Pale conjunctiva and muddy sclera
- Abdomen is nontender and bowel sounds are normal
- Slight tenderness in left lumbar region
- No past history of surgery
- No nausea, vomiting, diarrhea, constipation, or bloating

Relevant Lab Findings

- RBC count: 3.2×10^{12}/L (low); hemoglobin: 10.2 g/dL (low); hematocrit: 30% (low)
- Urine culture shows >100,000 CFU/mL of E. coli sensitive to ciprofloxacin form within 48 hours
- Nephrogram shows a large amount of uptake in the right kidney ("prompt nephrogram") but a delay of uptake in the left kidney ("delayed nephrogram")
- A 5-minute delayed nephrogram shows a massively dilated pelvicalyceal system with blunting of the calyces

Diagnosis

- Ureteropelvic junction (UPJ) obstruction: UPJ obstruction is the most common obstructive lesion in childhood. Congenital UPJ obstruction most often results from an aperistaltic segment of the ureter due to abnormal smooth muscle bundles or smooth muscle replacement with connective tissue. In addition, UPJ obstruction may be due to the absence of interstitial cells of Cajal that create a basal electrical rhythm leading to contraction of smooth muscle cells (i.e., peristalsis). UPJ obstruction may also be caused by kinks or valves produced by infoldings of ureteral mucosa and smooth muscle layer.

Chapter **9**

Female Reproductive System

I The Indifferent Embryo

A. The genotype of the embryo (46,XX or 46,XY) is established at fertilization.

B. **DURING WEEKS 1–6,** the embryo remains in a sexually indifferent or undifferentiated stage. This means that genetically female embryos and genetically male embryos are phenotypically indistinguishable.

C. **DURING WEEK 7,** the indifferent embryo begins phenotypic sexual differentiation.

D. **BY WEEK 12,** female or male characteristics of the external genitalia can be recognized.

E. **BY WEEK 20,** phenotypic differentiation is complete.

F. Phenotypic sexual differentiation is determined by the ***Sry* gene** located on the short arm of the **Y chromosome** and may result in individuals with a **female phenotype**, an **intersex phenotype**, or a **male phenotype**. The *Sry* gene encodes for a protein called **testes-determining factor (TDF)**.

G. As the indifferent gonad develops into the testes, Leydig cells and Sertoli cells differentiate to produce **testosterone** and **Müllerian inhibiting factor (MIF)**, respectively. In the presence of TDF, testosterone, and MIF, the indifferent embryo will be directed to the male phenotype. In the absence of TDF, testosterone, and MIF, the indifferent embryo will be directed to the female phenotype.

II Development of the Gonads

A. THE OVARY

1. The **intermediate mesoderm** forms a longitudinal elevation along the dorsal body wall called the **urogenital ridge**, which later forms the **gonadal ridge.**
2. **Primary sex cords** develop from the gonadal ridge and incorporate primordial germ cells (XX genotype), which migrate into the gonad from the wall of the yolk sac. Primary sex cords extend into the medulla and develop into the **rete ovarii**, which eventually degenerates.
3. **Secondary sex cords** develop and incorporate primordial germ cells as a thin **tunica albuginea** forms.
4. The secondary sex cords break apart and form isolated cell clusters called **primordial follicles**, which contain **primary oocytes** surrounded by a layer of **simple squamous cells.**

B. RELATIVE DESCENT OF THE OVARIES

1. The ovaries originally develop within the abdomen but later undergo a relative descent into the pelvis as a result of disproportionate growth.
2. The **gubernaculum** may also play a role. The gubernaculum is a band of fibrous tissue along the posterior wall that extends from the medial pole of the ovary to the uterus at the junction of the uterine tubes, forming the **ovarian ligament**. The gubernaculum then continues into the labia majora, forming the **round ligament of the uterus**.

III Development of Genital Ducts (Figure 9-1)

A. PARAMESONEPHRIC (MÜLLERIAN) DUCTS

1. The cranial portions of the paramesonephric ducts develop into the **uterine tubes**.
2. The caudal portions of the paramesonephric ducts fuse in the midline to form the **uterovaginal primordium** and thereby bring together two peritoneal folds called the **broad ligament**.
3. The uterovaginal primordium develops into the **uterus**, **cervix**, and **superior 1/3 of the vagina**.
4. The paramesonephric ducts project into the dorsal wall of the cloaca and induce the formation of the **sinovaginal bulbs**. The sinovaginal bulbs fuse to form the solid **vaginal plate**, which canalizes and develops into the **inferior two-thirds of the vagina**.
5. Vestigial remnants of the paramesonephric duct may be found in the adult female and are called the **hydatid of Morgagni**.

B. MESONEPHRIC (WOLFFIAN) DUCTS AND TUBULES

1. The mesonephric ducts develop in the female as part of the urinary system because these ducts are critical in the formation of the definitive metanephric kidney. However, they degenerate in the female after formation of the metanephric kidney.
2. Vestigial remnants of the mesonephric ducts may be found in the adult female, called the **appendix vesiculosa** and **Gartner's duct**.
3. Vestigial remnants of the mesonephric tubules, called the **epoophoron** and the **paroophoron**, may be found in the adult female.

IV Development of the Primordia of External Genitalia (Figure 9-2)

A. A proliferation of mesoderm around the cloacal membrane causes the overlying ectoderm to rise up so that three structures are visible externally, which include the **phallus**, **urogenital folds**, and **labioscrotal swellings**.

B. The phallus forms the **clitoris** (**glans clitoris**, **corpora cavernosa clitoris**, and **vestibular bulbs**).

C. The urogenital folds form the **labia minora**.

D. The labioscrotal swellings form the **labia majora** and **mons pubis**.

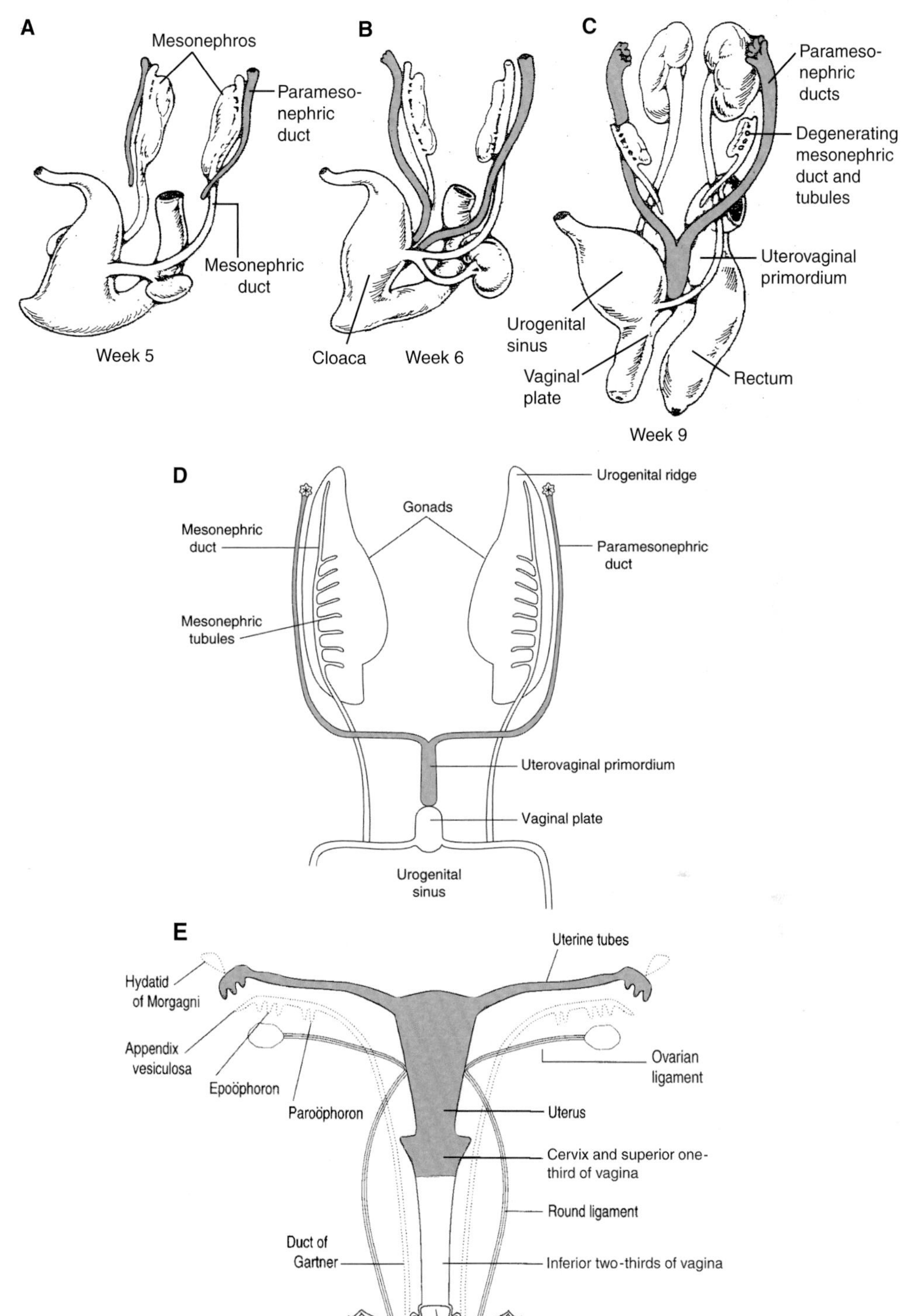

● **Figure 9-1 (A–C) Lateral view of the embryo. (A)** At week 5, paired paramesonephric ducts (*shaded*) begin to form along the lateral surface of the urogenital ridge at the mesonephros and grow in close association to the mesonephric duct. **(B)** At week 6, the paramesonephric ducts grow caudally and project into the dorsal wall of the cloaca and induce the formation of the sinovaginal bulbs (*not shown*). The mesonephric ducts continue to prosper. **(C)** At week 9, the caudal portions of the paramesonephric ducts fuse in the midline to form the uterovaginal primordium, and the sinovaginal bulbs fuse to form the vaginal plate at the urogenital sinus. During this time period, the mesonephric duct and mesonephric tubules both degenerate in the female. **(D)** Genital ducts in the indifferent embryo. **(E)** Female components and vestigial remnants (*dotted lines*) at birth.

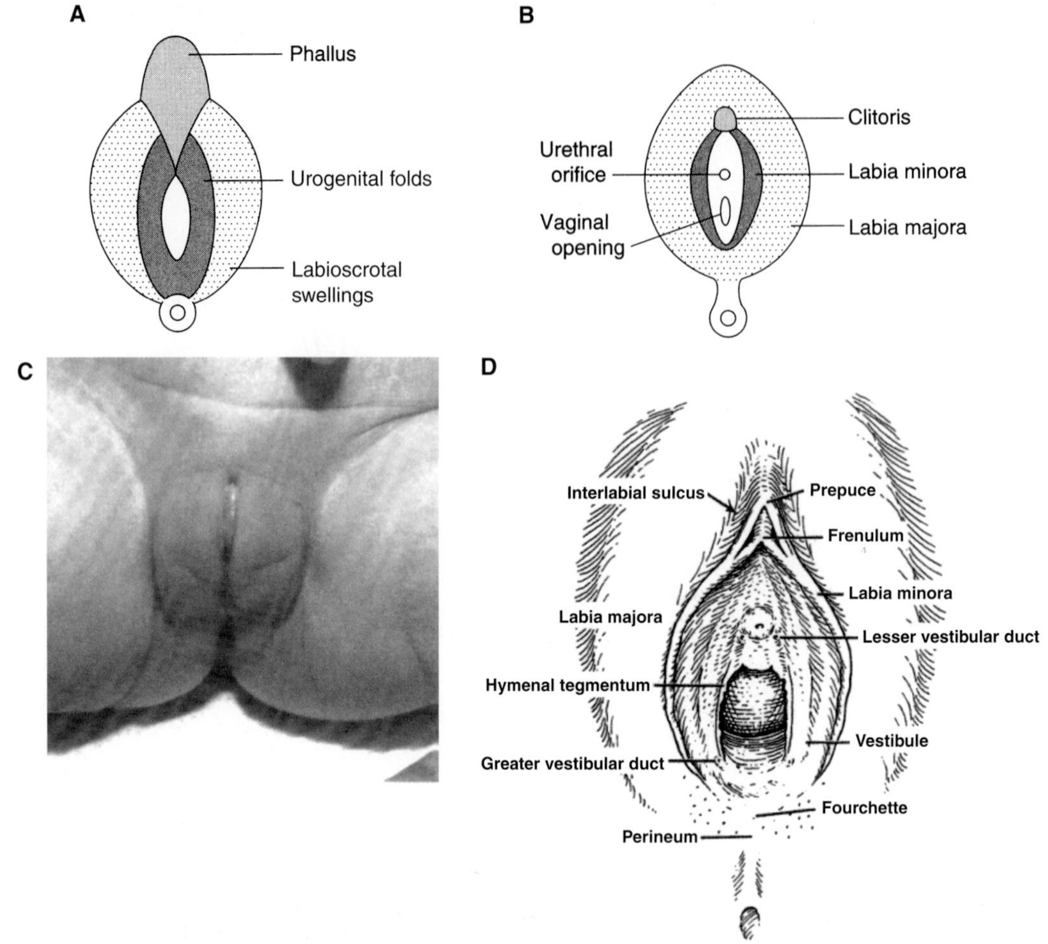

● **Figure 9-2** (A, B) Diagrams indicating the differentiation of the phallus, urogenital folds, and labioscrotal swellings in the female. **(A)** At week 5. **(B)** At birth. **(C)** Appearance of normal female genitalia at birth. **(D)** Diagram of the gross anatomy of the vulvar region in the adult female.

V Clinical Considerations

A. VESTIGIAL REMNANTS (FIGURE 9-3). The location of various cysts within the female reproductive tract is related to vestigial remnants of the genital ducts. Figure 9-3 shows the following cysts: (1) **Hydatid cyst of Morgagni** arises from the hydatid of Morgagni, which is a remnant of the paramesonephric duct. (2) **Kobelt's cyst** arises from the appendix vesiculosa, which is a remnant of the mesonephric duct. (3) **Cyst of the epoophoron** (type II) arises from the epoophoron, which is a remnant of the mesonephric tubules. (4) **Cyst of the paroophoron** arises from the paroophoron, which is a remnant of the mesonephric

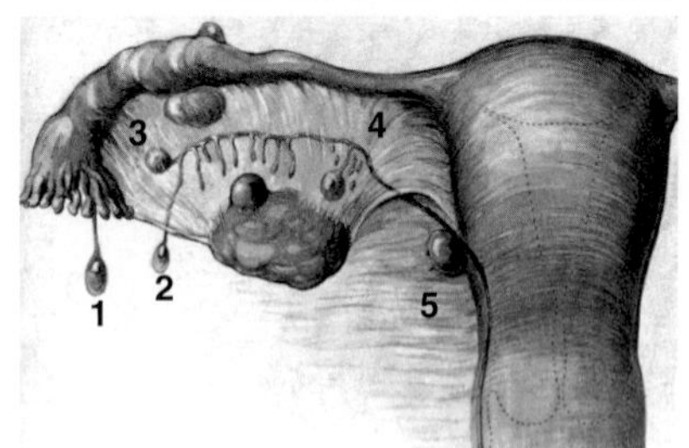

● **Figure 9-3 Vestigial remnants.**

tubules. (5) **Gartner's duct** cyst arises from the duct of Gartner, which is a remnant of the mesonephric duct.

B. UTERINE ANOMALIES

1. **Müllerian hypoplasia or agenesis anomalies (class I) (Figure 9-4)** involving the paramesonephric ducts can result in vaginal, cervical, uterine, uterine tube, or combined anomalies. Figure 9-4 shows (1) lower vagina agenesis, (2) cervix agenesis, (3) uterus and cervix hypoplasia, and (4) uterine tube agenesis.

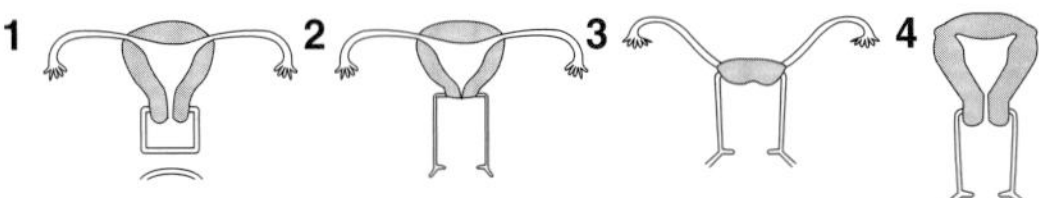

● **Figure 9-4 Müllerian hypoplasia and agenesis anomalies. Class I.**

2. **Unicornuate uterus anomalies (class II) (Figure 9-5)** occur when one paramesonephric duct fails to develop or incompletely develops. Figure 9-5 shows (1) unicornuate uterus with a communicating rudimentary horn, (2) unicornuate uterus with a noncommunicating rudimentary horn, (3) unicornuate uterus with a rudimentary horn containing no uterine cavity, and (4) unicornuate uterus. The hysterosalpingography (HSG) shows a single lenticular-shaped uterine canal with no evidence of a rudimentary right horn. There is filling of the left uterine tube.

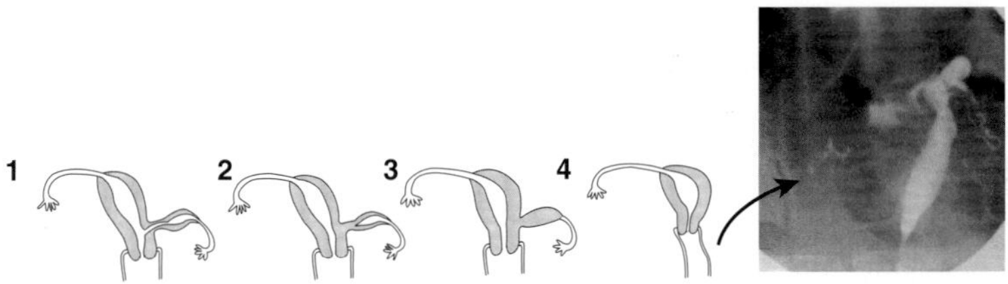

● **Figure 9-5 Unicornuate anomalies.** Class II.

3. **Didelphys (double uterus) anomalies (class III) (Figure 9-6)** occur when there is a complete lack of fusion of the paramesonephric ducts. Figure 9-6 shows the following: (1) Didelphys with normal vagina. A HSG shows a double uterus with a single normal vagina (top panel). (2) Didelphys with complete vaginal septum. A HSG shows a double uterus with a double vagina due to vaginal septum (bottom panel). This 17-year-old girl uses two tampons during menses.

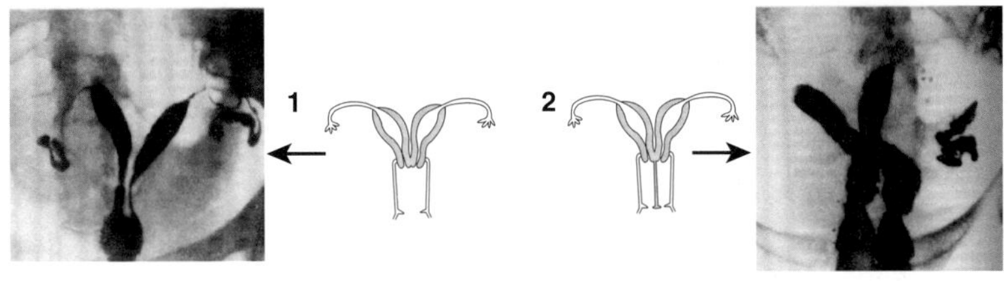

● **Figure 9-6 Didelphys (double uterus) anomalies.** Class III.

4. **Bicornuate uterus anomalies (class IV) (Figure 9-7)** occur when there is partial fusion of the paramesonephric ducts. Figure 9-7 shows (1) bicornuate uterus with complete division down to the internal os, and (2) bicornuate uterus with partial division. A HSG shows the uterine cavity partitioned into two channels.

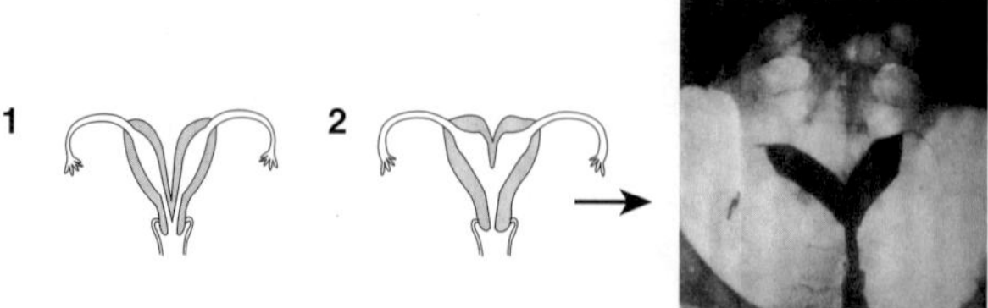

● **Figure 9-7 Bicornuate anomalies.**

5. **Septate uterus anomalies (class V) (Figure 9-8)** occur when the medial walls of the caudal portion of the paramesonephric ducts partially or completely fail to resorb. Figure 9-8 shows (1) septate uterus with complete septum down to the external os, and (2) septate uterus with partial septum.

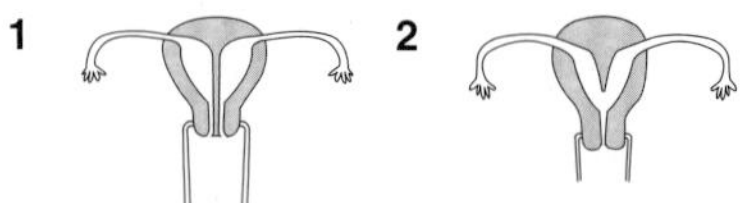

● **Figure 9-8 Septate uterus anomalies.** Class V.

6. **Diethylstilbestrol-related anomalies (Figure 9-9)**. Diethylstilbestrol (DES) was used until 1970 in the treatment of abortions, preeclampsia, diabetes, and preterm labor. For a female offspring exposed to DES in utero, an increased incidence of vaginal and cervical adenocarcinoma has been documented. In addition, many uterine anomalies, including T-shaped uterus, have been observed. The HSG in Figure 9-9 shows a T-shaped uterus. The second HSG shows a normal female reproductive tract for comparison. Arrowheads show uterine tubes; C indicates a catheter in the cervical canal.

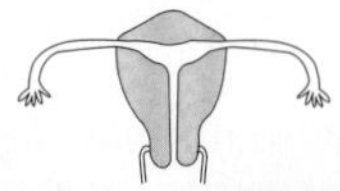

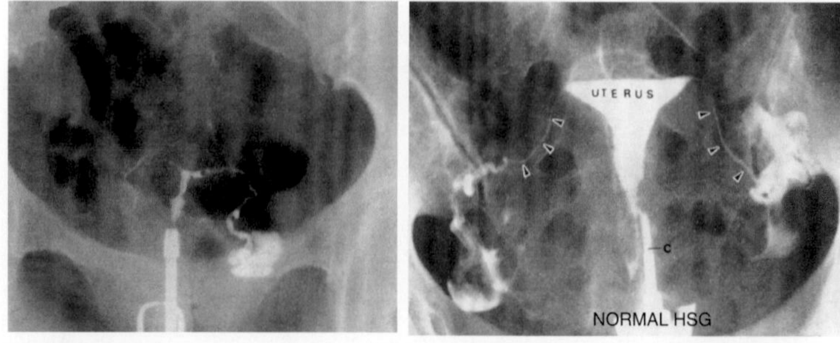

● **Figure 9-9 Diethylstilbestrol (DES)-related uterus anomalies.** Arrowheads show uterine tubes; C indicates a catheter in the cervical canal. HSG = hysterosalpingography.

Case Study

A woman comes in with her 16-year-old daughter and states that her daughter "has not had a menstrual period yet." The daughter says that she is not sexually active and that she is not on any form of birth control.

Differentials

- Turner syndrome, congenital adrenal hyperplasia, pituitary tumor, pituitary insufficiency

Relevant Physical Exam Findings

- Ambiguous genitalia
- Amenorrhea
- Early appearance of axillary and pubic hair

Relevant Lab Findings

- Elevated urinary 17-ketosteroids
- Elevated serum dehydroepiandrosterone (DHEA) sulfate
- Normal or decreased 17-hydroxycorticosteroids
- Genetic testing reveals 46,XX genotype
- Computed tomography (CT) head scan reveals no sign of tumor

Diagnosis

- Female pseudointersexuality (congenital adrenal hyperplasia) occurs when a woman has a 21-hydroxylase deficiency, which prevents the formation of aldosterone and cortisol and shifts the hormone precursors to form male sex hormones. Although Turner syndrome is also a cause of primary amenorrhea, individuals with Turner syndrome have a 45, XO genotype. A pituitary tumor can be excluded due to negative CT scan findings. A pituitary insufficiency can be ruled out because adrenal gland hormone production is present, which indicates that pituitary gland signaling to the adrenal glands is intact.

Chapter 10
Male Reproductive System

I The Indifferent Embryo

A. The genotype of the embryo (46,XX or 46,XY) is established at fertilization.

B. DURING WEEKS 1–6, the embryo remains in a sexually indifferent or undifferentiated stage. This means that genetically female embryos and genetically male embryos are phenotypically indistinguishable.

C. DURING WEEK 7, the indifferent embryo begins phenotypic sexual differentiation.

D. BY WEEK 12, female or male characteristics of the external genitalia can be recognized.

E. BY WEEK 20, phenotypic differentiation is complete.

F. Phenotypic sexual differentiation is determined by the ***Sry* gene** located on the short arm of the Y chromosome and may result in individuals with a **female phenotype**, an **intersex phenotype**, or a **male phenotype**. The *Sry* gene encodes for a protein called **testes-determining factor (TDF)**.

G. As the indifferent gonad develops into the testes, Leydig cells and Sertoli cells differentiate to produce **testosterone** and **Müllerian inhibiting factor (MIF)**, respectively. In the presence of TDF, testosterone, and MIF, the indifferent embryo will be directed to the male phenotype. In the absence of TDF, testosterone, and MIF, the indifferent embryo will be directed to the female phenotype.

II Development of the Gonads

A. THE TESTES

1. The **intermediate mesoderm** forms a longitudinal elevation along the dorsal body wall called the **urogenital ridge**, which later forms the **gonadal ridge**.
2. **Primary sex cords** develop from the gonadal ridge and incorporate primordial germ cells (XY genotype), which migrate into the gonad from the wall of the yolk sac. The primary sex cords extend into the medulla of the gonad and lose their connection with the surface epithelium as the thick **tunica albuginea** forms. The primary sex cords form the **seminiferous cords**, **tubuli recti**, and **rete testes**.
3. Seminiferous cords consist of **primordial germ cells** and **sustentacular (Sertoli) cells**, which secrete **MIF**.
4. The mesoderm between the seminiferous cords gives rise to the **interstitial (Leydig) cells**, which secrete **testosterone**.

5. The seminiferous cords remain as solid cords until puberty, when they acquire a lumen and are then called **seminiferous tubules.**

B. RELATIVE DESCENT OF THE TESTES

1. The testes originally develop within the abdomen but later undergo a relative descent into the scrotum as a result of disproportionate growth of the upper abdominal region away from the pelvic region.
2. The **gubernaculum** may also play a role. The gubernaculum is a band of fibrous tissue along the posterior wall that extends from the caudal pole of the testes to the scrotum. Remnants of the gubernaculum in the adult male serve to anchor the testes within the scrotum.
3. The peritoneum evaginates alongside the gubernaculum to form the **processus vaginalis.** Later in development, most of the processus vaginalis is obliterated except at its distal end, which remains as a peritoneal sac called the **tunica vaginalis** of the testes.

III Development of the Genital Ducts (Figure 10-1)

A. PARAMESONEPHRIC (MÜLLERIAN) DUCTS

1. The cranial portions of the paramesonephric ducts run parallel to the mesonephric ducts.
2. The caudal portions of the paramesonephric ducts fuse in the midline to form the uterovaginal primordium.
3. Under the influence of MIF, the cranial portions of the paramesonephric ducts and the uterovaginal primordium regress.
4. Vestigial remnants of the paramesonephric duct (called the **appendix testis**) may be found in the adult male.

B. MESONEPHRIC (WOLFFIAN) DUCTS AND TUBULES

1. The mesonephric ducts develop in the male as part of the urinary system because these ducts are critical in the formation of the definitive metanephric kidney.
2. The mesonephric ducts then proceed to additionally form the **epididymis, ductus deferens, seminal vesicle,** and **ejaculatory duct.**
3. A few mesonephric tubules in the region of the testes form the **efferent ductules** of the testes.
4. Vestigial remnants of the mesonephric duct (called the **appendix epididymis**) may be found in the adult male. Vestigial remnants of mesonephric tubules (called the **paradidymis**) also may be found in the adult male.

IV Development of the Primordia of External Genitalia (Figure 10-2)

A. A proliferation of mesoderm around the cloacal membrane causes the overlying ectoderm to rise up so that three structures are visible externally: the **phallus, urogenital folds,** and **labioscrotal swellings.**

B. The phallus forms the **penis (glans penis, corpora cavernosa penis, and corpus spongiosum penis).**

C. The urogenital folds form the **ventral aspect of the penis** (i.e., **penile raphe**).

D. The labioscrotal swellings form the **scrotum.**

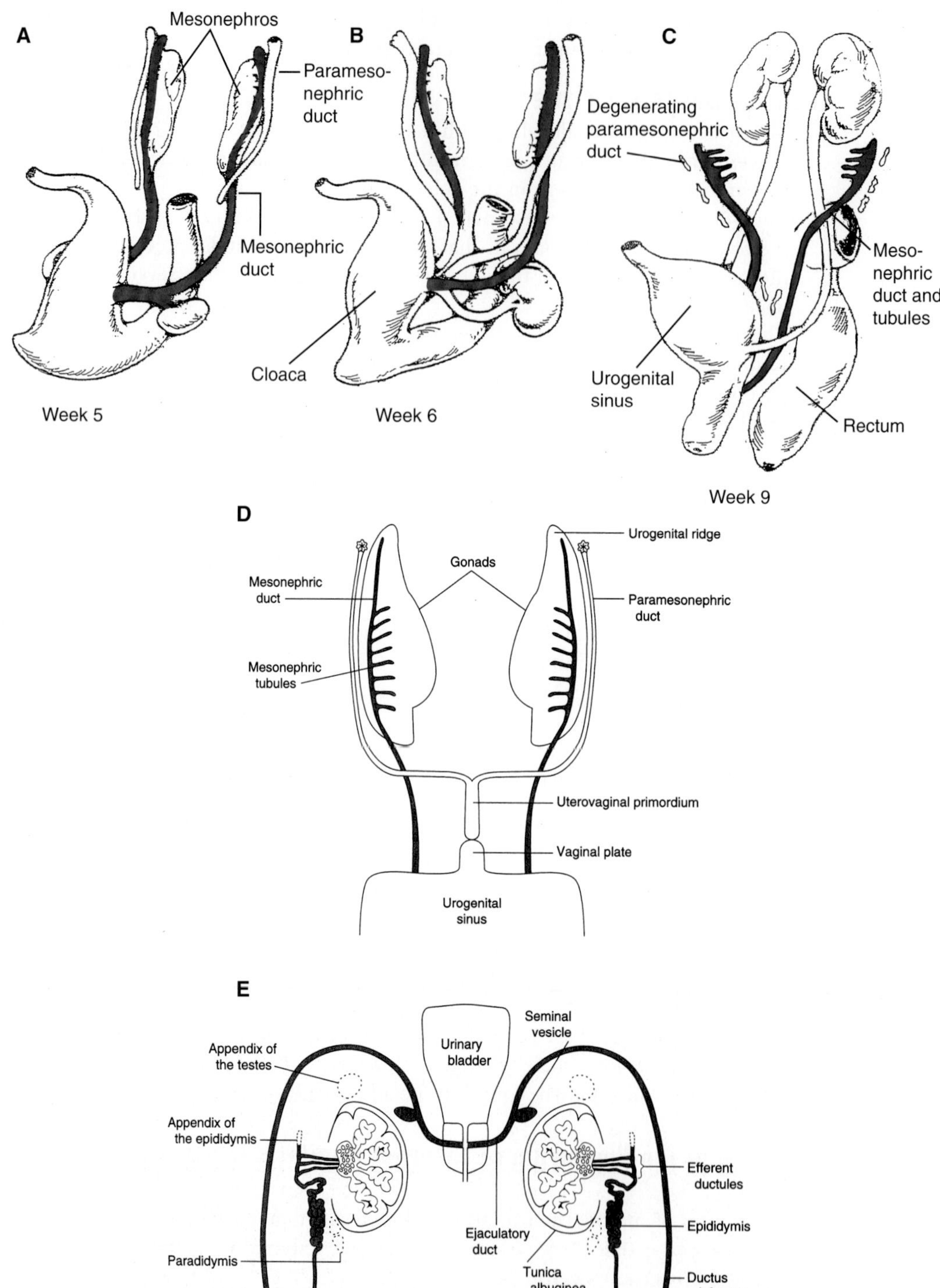

● **Figure 10-1 (A–C) Lateral view of the embryo. (A)** At week 5, paired paramesonephric ducts begin to form along the lateral surface of the urogenital ridge at the mesonephros and grow in close association with the mesonephric duct (*shaded*). **(B)** At week 6, the paramesonephric ducts grow caudally and project into the dorsal wall of the cloaca and induce the formation of the sinovaginal bulbs (*not shown*). The mesonephric ducts continue to prosper. **(C)** At week 9, the mesonephric ducts and mesonephric tubules establish contact with the testes and develop into definitive adult structures. During this time period, the paramesonephric ducts degenerate in the male. **(D)** Genital ducts in the indifferent embryo. **(E)** Male components and vestigial remnants (*dotted lines*). The mesonephric ducts/tubules and their derivatives are shaded.

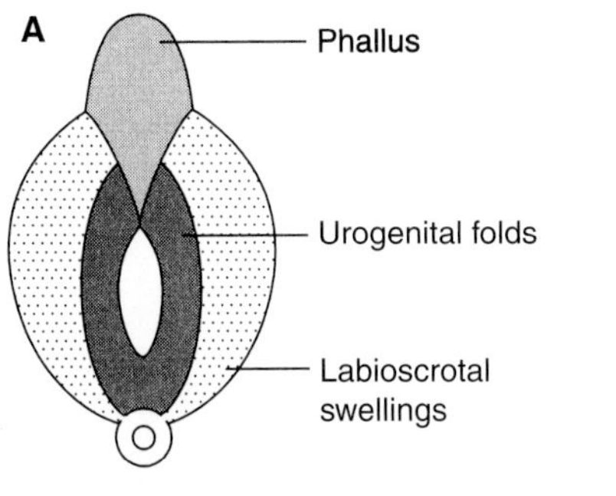

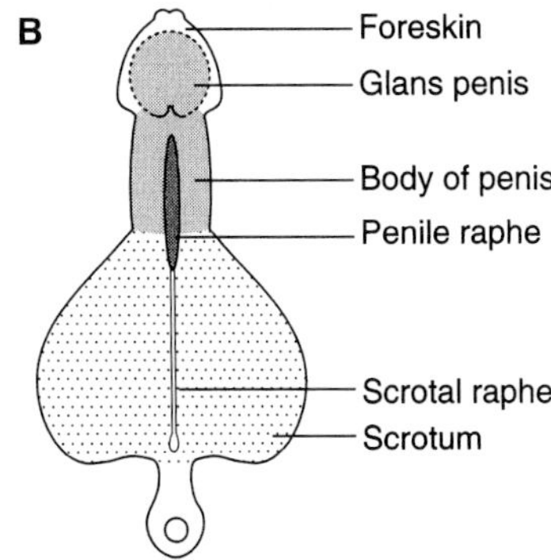

● **Figure 10-2 (A, B)** Diagrams indicating the differentiation of the phallus, urogenital folds, and labioscrotal swellings in the male. **(A)** At week 5. **(B)** At birth.

V Clinical Considerations

A. MALE ANOMALIES

1. **Hypospadias (Figure 10-3)** occurs when the urethral folds fail to fuse completely, resulting in the external urethral orifice opening onto the ventral surface of the penis. Hypospadias is generally associated with a poorly developed penis that curves ventrally, known as **chordee**. The left photograph in Figure 10-3 shows hypospadias with the urethral opening on the ventral surface (arrow). The right photograph shows chordee, where the penis is poorly developed and bowed ventrally.

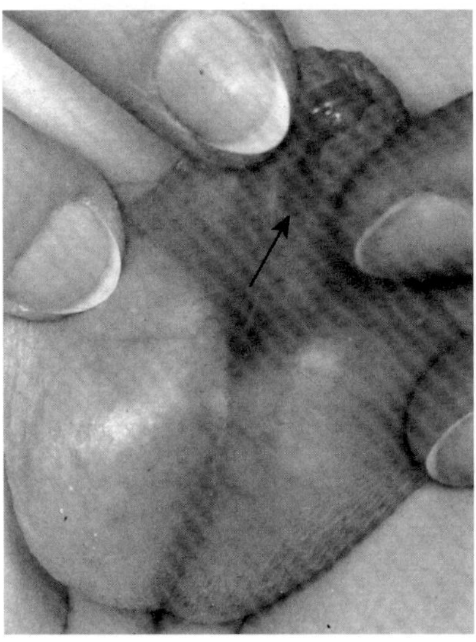

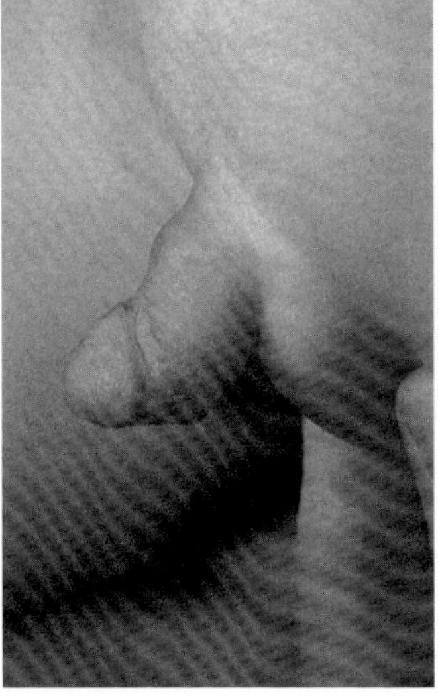

● **Figure 10-3 Hypospadias.**

2. **Epispadias (Figure 10-4)** occurs when the external urethral orifice opens onto the dorsal surface of the penis. It is generally associated with **exstrophy of the bladder**. Figure 10-4 shows epispadias with the urethral opening on the dorsal surface of the penis (arrows), whereby the penis is almost split in half.
3. **Undescended testes (cryptorchidism) (Figure 10-5)** occurs when the testes fail to descend into the scrotum. Descent of the testes is evident within 3 months after birth. Bilateral cryptorchidism results in **sterility**. The undescended testes may be found in the abdominal cavity or in the inguinal canal and are surgically removed because they pose an increased risk of testicular cancer. Figure 10-5 shows cryptorchidism in which both testes have not descended into the scrotal sac. The arrow points to one of the undescended testes.
4. **Hydrocele of the testes (Figure 10-6)** occurs when a small patency of the processus vaginalis remains so that peritoneal fluid can flow into the processus vaginalis, which results in a fluid-filled cyst near the testes. This demonstrates as a scrotal enlargement that transilluminates due to persistence of tunica vaginalis. Figure 10-6 shows a bilateral hydrocele.
5. **Congenital inguinal hernia** occurs when a large patency of the processus vaginalis remains so that a loop of intestine may herniate into the scrotum or labia majora. It is most common in males and is generally associated with cryptorchidism.

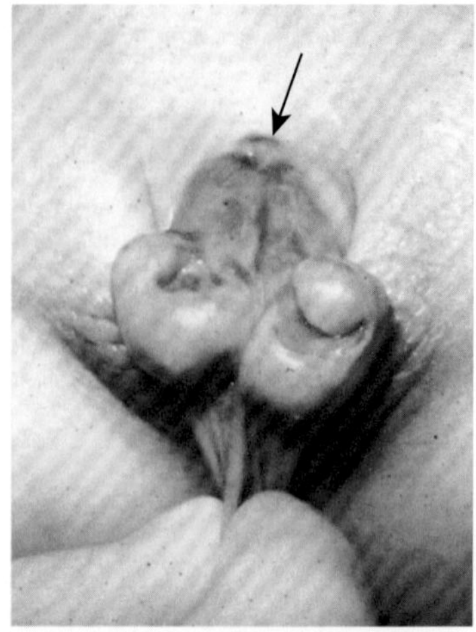

● **Figure 10-4 Epispadias.**

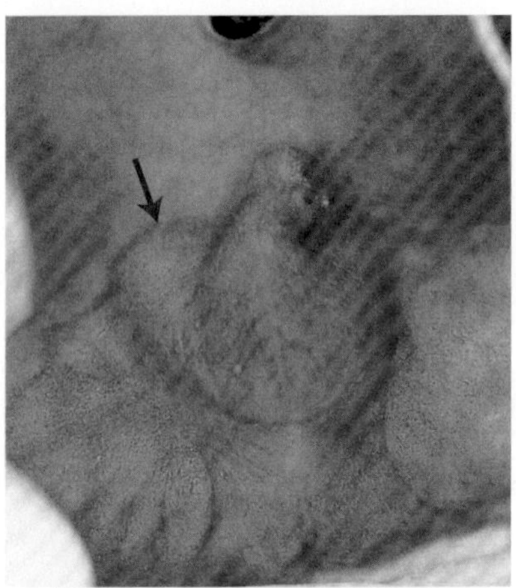

● **Figure 10-5 Undescended testes (cryptorchidism).**

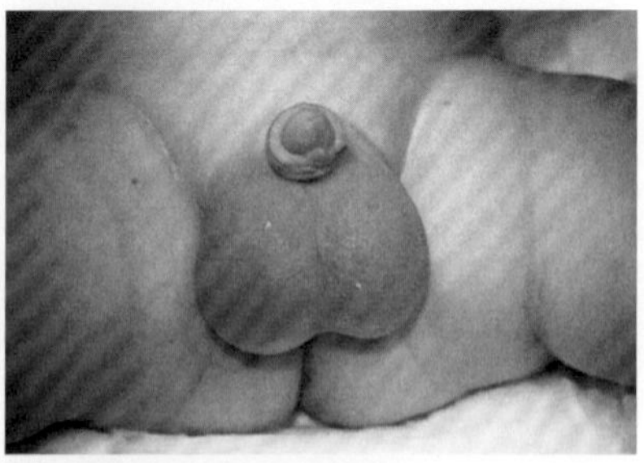

● **Figure 10-6 Hydrocele of the testes.**

B. INTERSEX ANOMALIES

1. **Intersexuality.** Because the early embryo goes through an indifferent stage, events may occur whereby a fetus does not progress toward either of the two usual phenotypes, but gets caught in an intermediate stage known as intersexuality. Intersexuality is classified according to the histological appearance of the **gonad** and **ambiguous genitalia**. **True intersexuality** occurs when an individual has both ovarian and testicular tissue (ovotestes) histologically, ambiguous genitalia, and a 46,XX genotype. True intersexuality is a rare condition whose cause is poorly understood.
2. **Female pseudointersexuality (FP) (Figure 10-7)** occurs when an individual has only ovarian tissue histologically and masculinization of the female external genitalia. These individuals have a **46,XX genotype.** FP is most often observed clinically in association with a condition in which the fetus produces an **excess of androgens** (e.g., **congenital adrenal hyperplasia** [CAH]). CAH is caused most commonly by mutations in genes for enzymes involved in adrenocortical steroid biosynthesis (e.g., **21-hydroxylase deficiency, 11β-hydroxylase deficiency**). **In 21-hydroxylase deficiency (90% of all cases)**, there is virtually no synthesis of the cortisol or aldosterone so that intermediates are funneled into androgen biosynthesis, thereby elevating androgen levels. The elevated levels of androgens lead to **masculinization of a female fetus.** FP produces the following clinical findings: mild clitoral enlargement, complete labioscrotal fusion with a phalloid organ, or macrogenitosomia (in the male fetus). Because cortisol cannot be synthesized, negative feedback to the adenohypophysis does not occur, so adrenocorticotropic hormone (ACTH) continues to stimulate the adrenal cortex, resulting in adrenal hyperplasia. Because aldosterone cannot be synthesized, the patient presents with **hyponatremia ("salt-wasting")** with accompanying **dehydration** and **hyperkalemia.** Treatment includes immediate infusion of intravenous saline and long-term steroid hormone replacement, both cortisol and mineralocorticoids (9α fludrocortisone). Figure 10-7 shows a patient (XX genotype; female) with FP due to CAH. The masculinization of female external genitalia is apparent with fusion of the labia majora and enlarged clitoris (see arrow to inset).

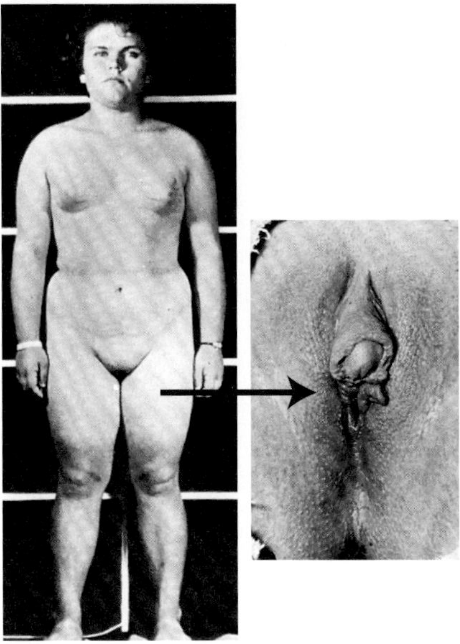

● **Figure 10-7 Female pseudointersexuality.**

3. **Male pseudointersexuality (MP) (Figure 10-8)** occurs when an individual has only testicular tissue histologically and various stages of stunted development of the male external genitalia. These individuals have a **46,XY genotype**. MP is most often observed clinically in association with a condition in which the fetus produces a **lack of androgens (and MIF)**. This is caused most commonly by mutations in genes for androgen steroid biosynthesis (e.g., **5α-reductase 2 deficiency** or **17β-hydroxysteroid dehydrogenase [HSD] deficiency**). Normally, 5α-reductase 2 catalyzes the conversion of testosterone (T) → dihydrotestosterone (DHT), and 17β-HSD3 catalyzes the conversion of androstenedione → testosterone. An increased T:DHT ratio is diagnostic (normal = 5; 5α-reductase 2 deficiency = 20–60). The reduced levels of androgens lead to the feminization of a male fetus. MP produces the following clinical findings: underdevelopment of the penis, scrotum (microphallus, hypospadias, and bifid scrotum), and prostate gland. The epididymis, ductus deferens, seminal vesicle, and ejaculatory duct are normal. These clinical findings have led to the inference that DHT is essential in the development of the penis and scrotum (external genitalia) and prostate gland in a genotypic XY fetus. At puberty, these individuals demonstrate a striking virilization. Figure 10-8 shows a patient (XY genotype; male) with MP. The stunted development of male external genitalia is apparent. The stunted external genitalia fooled the parents and physician at birth into thinking that this XY infant was actually a girl. In fact, this child was raised as a girl (note the pigtails). As this child neared puberty, testosterone levels increased and clitoral enlargement ensued. This alarmed the parents, and the child was brought in for clinical evaluation.

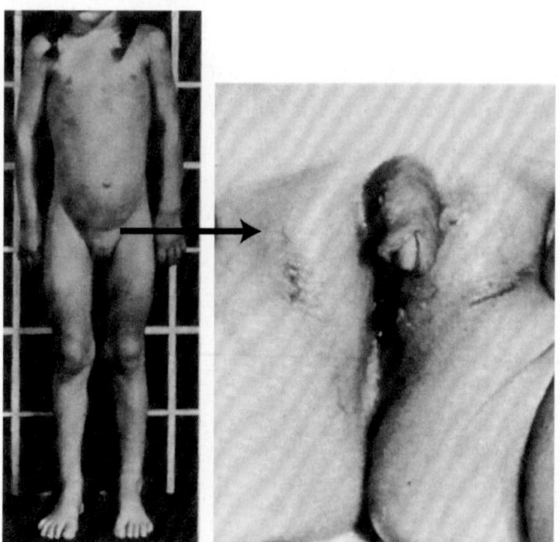

● **Figure 10-8 Male pseudointersexuality.**

4. **Complete androgen insensitivity (CAIS; or testicular feminization syndrome) (Figure 10-9)** occurs when a fetus with a 46,XY genotype develops testes and female external genitalia with a rudimentary vagina; uterus and uterine tubes are generally absent. The testes may be found in the labia majora and are surgically removed to circumvent malignant tumor formation. These individuals present as normal-appearing females, and their psychosocial orientation is female despite their genotype. The most common cause is a mutation in the gene for the **androgen receptor.** Even though the developing male fetus is exposed to normal levels of androgens, the lack of androgen receptors renders the phallus, urogenital folds, and labioscrotal swellings unresponsive to androgens. Figure 10-9 shows a patient (XY genotype) with CAIS, in whom complete feminization of male external genitalia along with other secondary sex characteristics is apparent.

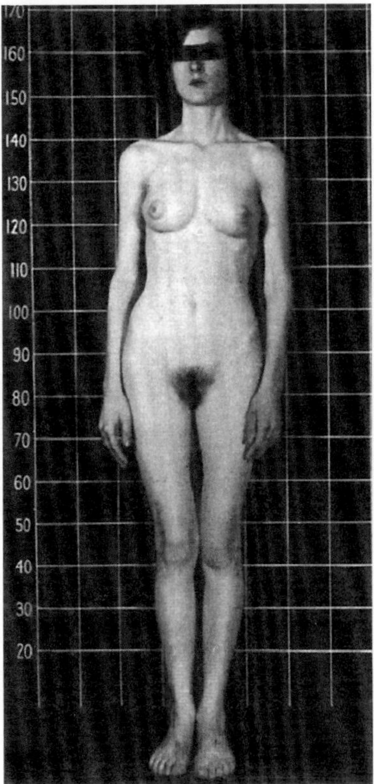

● **Figure 10-9 Complete androgen insensitivity (CAIS).**

 Summary Table of Female and Male Reproductive Systems Development (Table 10-1)

TABLE 10-1 FEMALE AND MALE REPRODUCTIVE SYSTEMS DEVELOPMENT

Adult Female	Indifferent Embryo	Adult Male
Ovary, ovarian follicles, rete ovarii	**Gonads**	Testes, seminiferous tubules, tubuli recti, rete testes, Leydig cells, Sertoli cells
Uterine tubes, uterus, cervix, superior 1/3 of vagina	**Paramesonephric duct**	—
Hydatid of Morgagni		*Appendix testes*
—	**Mesonephric duct**	Epididymis, ductus deferens, seminal vesicle, ejaculatory duct
Appendix vesiculosa, Gartner's duct		*Appendix epididymis*
—	**Mesonephric tubules**	Efferent ductules
Epoophoron, paroophoron		*Paradidymis*
Glans clitoris, corpora cavernosa clitoris, vestibular bulbs	**Phallus**	Glans penis, corpora cavernosa penis, corpus spongiosum
Labia minora	**Urogenital folds**	Ventral aspect of penis
Labia majora, mons pubis	**Labioscrotal swellings**	Scrotum
Ovarian ligament, round ligament of uterus	**Gubernaculum**	Gubernaculum testes
—	**Processus vaginalis**	Tunica vaginalis

Italics indicates vestigial structures.

Case Study

A concerned couple brings their 3-week-old son into your office, stating that they think something is wrong with their son's genital area. They noticed that his testicles appeared to be swollen when they were changing his diaper a week ago. They said that his scrotum felt like a "water-filled balloon." Neither parent could recall any traumatic episode with their son, saying that they have been very protective of him.

Differential

- Hydrocele, hematocele, inguinal hernia, obstruction within spermatic cord

Relevant Physical Exam Findings

- Enlarged scrotum that is nontender
- Testicles not immediately palpable
- No herniated bulge found
- Flashlight test through the enlarged area showed illumination

Relevant Lab Findings

- Negative blood on fluid collection
- Ultrasound confirm hydrocele

Diagnosis

- Hydrocele occurs when there is a patent tunica vaginalis. Peritoneal fluid drains from the abdomen through the tunica vaginalis. The fluid accumulates in the scrotum, becomes trapped, and causes the scrotum to enlarge. A hydrocele is usually harmless and in most cases resolves within a few months after birth. A hydrocele is normally treated only when there is discomfort or when the testicular blood supply is threatened. A hematocele could have also been considered, but a hematocele is typically due to trauma, and blood would have been seen on fluid collection. Inguinal hernias usually accompany hydroceles, but there was no bulge detected on physical examination. Obstruction within spermatic cord is usually seen in older men.

Chapter 11

Respiratory System

I Upper Respiratory System consists of the **nose**, **nasopharynx**, and **oropharynx**.

II Lower Respiratory System (Figure 11-1)

A. Consists of the **larynx**, **trachea**, **bronchi**, and **lungs**.

B. The first sign of development is the formation of the **respiratory (or laryngotracheal) diverticulum** in the ventral wall of the primitive foregut during week 4.

C. The distal end of the respiratory diverticulum enlarges to form the **lung bud**.

D. The lung bud divides into two **bronchial buds** that branch into the **main (primary)**, **lobar (secondary)**, **segmental (tertiary)**, **and subsegmental bronchi**.

E. The respiratory diverticulum initially is in open communication with the foregut, but eventually they become separated by indentations of mesoderm—the **tracheoesophageal folds**. When the tracheoesophageal folds fuse in the midline to form the **tracheoesophageal septum**, the foregut is divided into the **trachea** ventrally and **esophagus** dorsally.

III Development of the Trachea

A. FORMATION. The foregut is divided into the trachea ventrally and the esophagus dorsally by the **tracheoesophageal folds**, which fuse to form the **tracheoesophageal septum**.

B. CLINICAL CONSIDERATION. **Tracheoesophageal fistula (Figure 11-2)** is an abnormal communication between the trachea and esophagus that results from improper division of the foregut by the tracheoesophageal septum. It is generally associated with **esophageal atresia**, which will then result in **polyhydramnios**. Clinical features include: excessive accumulation of saliva or mucus in the nose and mouth; episodes

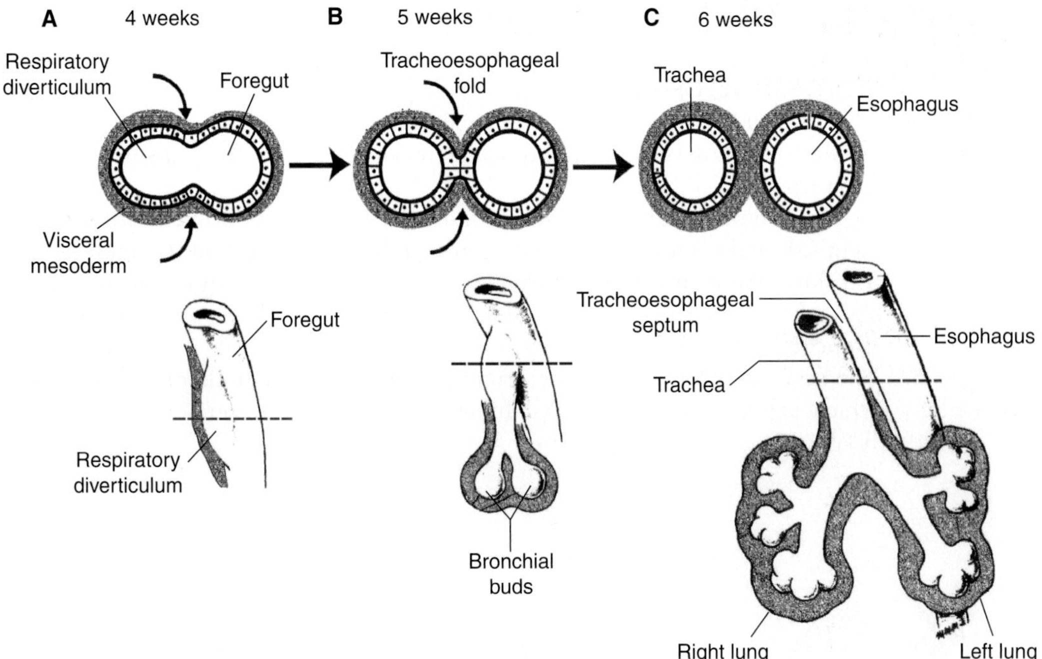

● **Figure 11-1 Development of the respiratory system.** At **(A)** 4 weeks, **(B)** 5 weeks, and **(C)** 6 weeks. Both lateral views and cross-sectional views are shown (dotted lines indicate the level of cross section). Note the relationship of the respiratory diverticulum and foregut. Curved arrows indicate the movement of the tracheoesophageal folds as the tracheoesophageal septum forms between the trachea and the esophagus.

of gagging and cyanosis after swallowing milk; abdominal distention after crying; and reflux of gastric contents into lungs, causing pneumonitis. Diagnostic features include inability to pass a catheter into the stomach and radiographs demonstrating air in the infant's stomach. Figure 11-2 shows an esophageal atresia with a tracheoesophageal fistula at the distal one-third end of the trachea. This is the most common type, occurring in 82% of cases. The anteroposterior (AP) radiograph of this malformation shows an enteric tube (arrow) coiled in the upper esophageal pouch. The air in the bowel indicates a distal tracheoesophageal fistula.

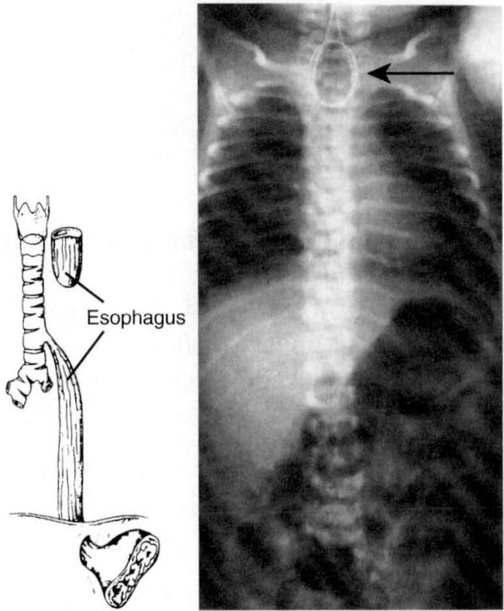

● **Figure 11-2 Esophageal atresia with a tracheoesophageal fistula at the distal one-third end of the trachea.**

IV Development of the Bronchi (Figure 11-3)

A. STAGES OF DEVELOPMENT

1. The lung bud divides into two **bronchial buds**.
2. In week 5 of development, bronchial buds enlarge to form **main (primary) bronchi**.
3. The main bronchi further subdivide into **lobar (secondary) bronchi** (three on the right side and two on the left side, corresponding to the lobes of the adult lung).
4. The lobar bronchi further subdivide into **segmental (tertiary) bronchi** (10 on the right side and 9 on the left side), which further subdivide into **subsegmental bronchi**.
5. The segmental bronchi are the primordia of the **bronchopulmonary segments**, which are morphologically and functionally separate respiratory units of the lung.

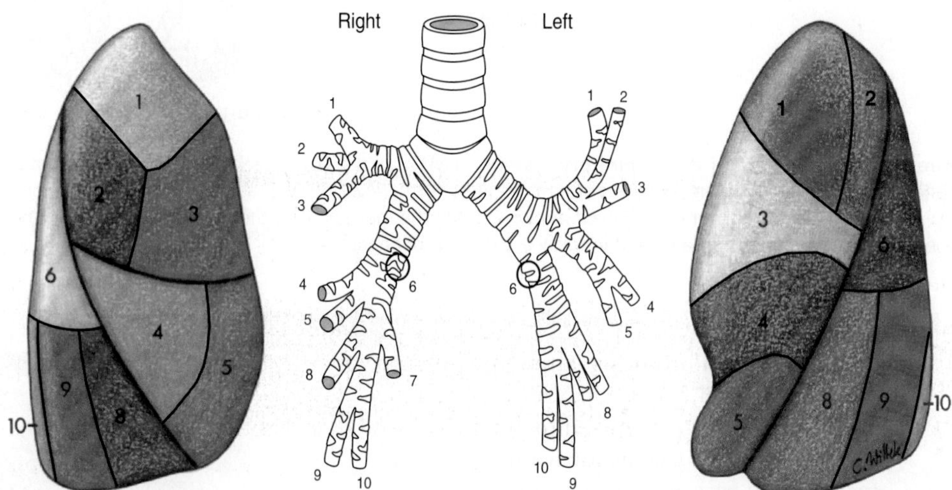

● **Figure 11-3 Distribution of bronchopulmonary segments and their relationship to the tracheobronchial tree.** Segmental bronchi of the right and left lungs are numbered. Right lung: 1–3: segmental bronchi that branch from the upper lobar bronchus; 4, 5: segmental bronchi that branch from the middle lobar bronchus; 6–10: segmental bronchi that branch from the lower lobar bronchus. Note that bronchopulmonary segment 7 is not represented on the outer costal surface of the right lung (segment 7 is located on the inner mediastinal surface). Left lung: 1–5: segmental bronchi that branch from the upper lobar bronchus; 6–10: segmental bronchi that branch from the lower lobar bronchus. Note that there is no segment 7 bronchus associated with the left lung.

B. CLINICAL CONSIDERATIONS

1. **Bronchopulmonary segment** is a segment of lung tissue supplied by a segmental (tertiary) bronchus. Surgeons can resect diseased lung tissue along bronchopulmonary segments rather than remove the entire lobe.

2. **Congenital lobar emphysema (CLE) (Figure 11-4)** is characterized by progressive overdistention of one of the upper lobes or the right middle lobe with **air**. The term *emphysema* is a misnomer because there is no destruction of the alveolar walls. Although the exact etiology is unknown, many cases involve **collapsed bronchi** due to **failure of bronchial cartilage formation.** In this situation, air can be inspired through collapsed bronchi but cannot be expired. During the first few days of life, fluid may be trapped in the involved lobe, producing an opaque, enlarged hemithorax. Later, the fluid is resorbed and the classic radiological appearance of an emphysematous lobe with generalized radiolucency (hyperlucent) is apparent. The expiratory AP radiograph in Figure 11-4 shows a hyperlucent area in the emphysematous right upper lobe due to air trapping.

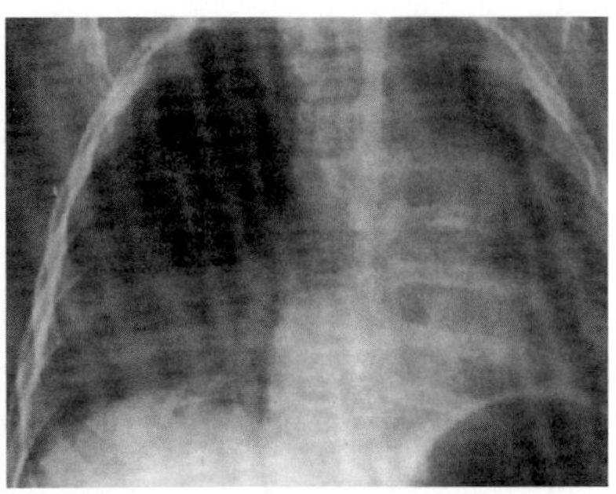

● **Figure 11-4 Congenital lobar emphysema.**

3. **Congenital bronchogenic cysts (Figure 11-5)** represent an abnormality in bronchial branching and may be found within the mediastinum (most commonly) or intrapulmonary. Intrapulmonary cysts are round, solitary, sharply marginated, and **fluid filled** and do not initially communicate with the tracheobronchial tree. Because intrapulmonary bronchogenic cysts contain fluid, they appear as water-density masses on chest radiographs. These cysts may become air filled as a result of infection or instrumentation. The AP radiograph in Figure 11-5 shows a large opaque area in the right upper lobe due to a fluid-filled cyst.

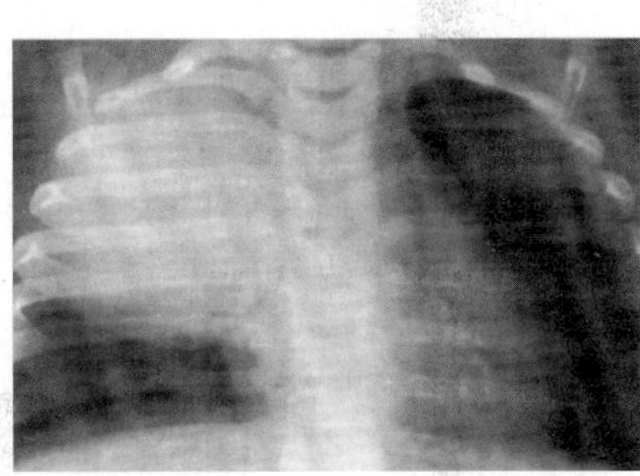

● **Figure 11-5 Congenital bronchogenic cyst.**

V Development of the Lungs

A. PERIODS OF DEVELOPMENT (TABLE 11-1)

1. The lung matures in a proximal–distal direction, beginning with the largest bronchi and proceeding outward. As a result, lung development is heterogeneous; proximal pulmonary tissue will be in a more advanced period of development than distal pulmonary tissue.
2. The periods of lung development include the **pseudoglandular period** (weeks 7–16), the **canalicular period** (weeks 16–24), the **terminal sac period** (week 24–birth), and the **alveolar period** (week 32–8 years).

TABLE 11-1 PERIODS OF LUNG DEVELOPMENT

Pseudoglandular period (weeks 7–16)

- The developing lung resembles an exocrine gland; numerous **endodermal tubules** are lined by a **simple columnar epithelium** and are surrounded by mesoderm containing a **modest capillary network**.
- Each endodermal tubule branches into 15–25 **terminal bronchioles**.
- **Respiration is not possible, and premature infants cannot survive**.

Canalicular period (weeks 16–24)

- The terminal bronchioles branch into three or more **respiratory bronchioles**.
- The respiratory bronchioles subsequently branch into three to six **alveolar ducts**.
- The terminal bronchioles, respiratory bronchioles, and alveolar ducts are now lined by a **simple cuboidal epithelium** and are surrounded by mesoderm containing a **prominent capillary network**.
- **Premature infants born before week 20 rarely survive**.

Terminal sac period (weeks 24–birth)

- The alveolar ducts bud off **terminal sacs**, which dilate and expand into the surrounding mesoderm.
- The terminal sacs are separated from each other by **primary septae**.
- The simple cuboidal epithelium within the terminal sacs differentiates into type **I pneumocytes** (thin, flat cells that make up part of the blood–air barrier) and **type II pneumocytes** (which secrete surfactant).
- The terminal sacs are surrounded by mesoderm containing a **rapidly proliferating capillary network**. The capillaries make intimate contact with the terminal sacs and thereby establish a **blood–air barrier** with the type I pneumocytes.
- **Premature infants born between weeks 25 and 28 can survive with intensive care**. Adequate vascularization and surfactant levels are the most important factors for the survival of premature infants.

Alveolar period (birth–8 years of age)

- The terminal sacs are partitioned by **secondary septae** to form adult **alveoli**. About 20–70 million alveoli are present at birth. About 300–400 million alveoli are present by 8 years of age.
- The major mechanism for the increase in the number of alveoli is the formation of secondary septae that partition existing alveoli.
- After birth, the increase in the size of the lung is due to an **increase in the number of respiratory bronchioles**.
- On chest radiographs, lungs of a newborn infant are denser than an adult lung because of the fewer mature alveoli.

B. CLINICAL CONSIDERATIONS

1. **Aeration at birth** is the replacement of lung liquid with air in the newborn's lungs. In the fetal state, the functional residual capacity (FRC) of the lung is filled with liquid secreted by fetal lung epithelium via Cl^- transport using cystic fibrosis transmembrane protein (CFTR). At birth, lung liquid is eliminated by a reduction in lung liquid secretion via Na^+ transport by type II pneumocytes and resorption into pulmonary capillaries (major route) and lymphatics (minor route). Lungs of a stillborn baby will sink when placed in water because they contain fluid rather than air.
2. **Pulmonary agenesis** is the complete absence of a lung or a lobe and its bronchi. This is a rare condition caused by failure of bronchial buds to develop. Unilateral pulmonary agenesis is compatible with life.
3. **Pulmonary aplasia** is the absence of lung tissue but the presence of a rudimentary bronchus.

4. **Pulmonary hypoplasia (PH)** is a poorly developed bronchial tree with abnormal histology. PH classically involves the right lung in association with right-sided obstructive congenital heart defects. PH can also be found in association with **congenital diaphragmatic hernia** (i.e., herniation of abdominal contents into the thorax), which compresses the developing lung. PH can also be found in association with **bilateral renal agenesis**, which causes an insufficient amount of amniotic fluid (oligohydramnios) to be produced, which in turn increases pressure on the fetal thorax.

5. **Hyaline membrane disease (HMD; Figure 11-6)** is caused by a deficiency or absence of **surfactant.** This surface-active agent is composed of **cholesterol** (50%), **dipalmitoylphosphatidylcholine** (DPPC; 40%), and **surfactant proteins A, B, and C** (10%) and coats the inside of alveoli to maintain alveolar patency. HMD is prevalent in premature infants (accounts for 50%–70% of deaths in premature infants), infants of diabetic mothers, infants who experienced fetal asphyxia or maternofetal hemorrhage (damages type II pneumocytes), and multiple-birth infants. Clinical signs include dyspnea, tachypnea, inspiratory retractions of chest wall, expiratory grunting, cyanosis, and nasal flaring. Treatments include administration of betamethasone (a corticosteroid) to the mother for several days before delivery (i.e., antenatal) to increase surfactant production, postnatal administration of an artificial surfactant solution, and postnatal high-frequency ventilation. HMD in premature infants cannot be discussed without mentioning **germinal matrix hemorrhage (GMH).** The germinal matrix is the site of proliferation of neuronal and glial precursors in the developing brain, which is located above the caudate nucleus, in the floor of the lateral ventricles, and in the caudo-thalamic groove. The germinal matrix also contains a rich network of fragile, thin-walled blood vessels. The brain of the premature infant lacks the ability to autoregulate the cerebral blood pressure. Consequently, increased arterial blood pressure in these blood vessels leads to rupture and hemorrhage into the germinal matrix. This leads to significant neurological sequelae, including cerebral palsy, mental retardation, and seizures. Antenatal corticosteroid administration

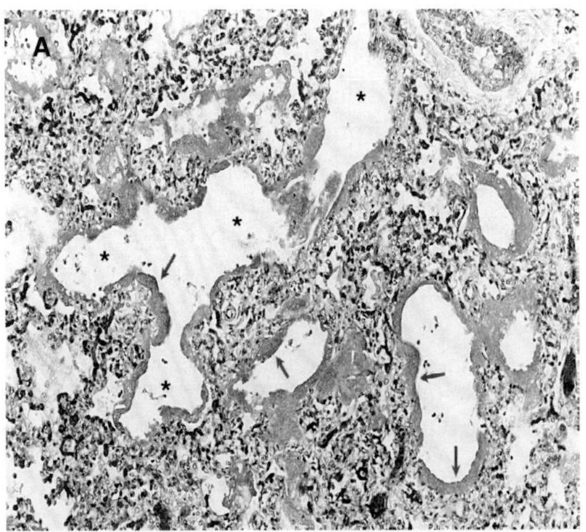

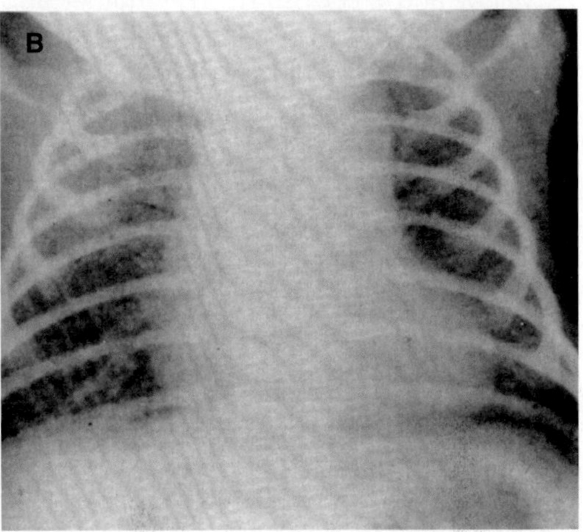

● **Figure 11-6 Hyaline Membrane Disease (HMD)**

has a clear role in reducing the incidence of GMH in premature infants. The light micrograph image in Figure 11-6 shows the pathological hallmarks of HMD: acinar atelectasis (i.e., collapse of the respiratory acinus, which includes the respiratory bronchioles, alveolar ducts, and alveoli), dilation of terminal bronchioles (*asterisks*), and deposition of an eosinophilic hyaline membrane material (arrows) that consists of fibrin and necrotic cells. The AP radiograph shows the radiological hallmarks of HMD: a bell-shaped thorax due to underaeration and reticulogranularity of the lungs caused by acinar atelectasis.

Case Study

A mother brings her 5-year-old son into your office on a follow-up visit. The child previously had a bout of pneumonia, and the mother remarks that the child has been coughing up "yellow and green stuff." The mother also remarks that he has had a number of coughs and colds that were just like this in the past. His chart is remarkable for cystic fibrosis. What is the most likely diagnosis?

Differential

- Asthma, bronchitis, pneumonia

Relevant Physical Exam Findings

- Foul-smelling greenish sputum with speckles of blood
- Orthopnea
- Fever

Relevant Lab Findings

- Spirometry shows a reduced ratio of forced expiratory volume in 1 second (FEV_1) to forced vital capacity (FVC).
- Chest X-ray shows multiple cysts, which have a "honeycomb" appearance.
- Computed tomography shows a dilation of bronchi.

Diagnosis

- Bronchiectasis

Chapter **12**

Head and Neck

I Pharyngeal Apparatus (Figure 12-1; Table 12-1)

consists of the **pharyngeal arches**, **pharyngeal pouches**, **pharyngeal grooves**, and **pharyngeal membranes**, which are first observed in week 4 of development and give the embryo its distinctive appearance. Pharyngeal arch 5 and pharyngeal pouch 5 completely regress in the human.

A. PHARYNGEAL ARCHES (1–4 AND 6; 5 REGRESSES IN HUMANS) contain **mesoderm** and **neural crest cells**. In general, the mesoderm differentiates into **muscles** and **arteries** (i.e., aortic arches 1–6), whereas neural crest cells differentiate into **bone** and **connective tissue**. In addition, each pharyngeal arch has a **cranial nerve** associated with it.

B. PHARYNGEAL POUCHES (1–4) are evaginations of endoderm that lines the foregut.

C. PHARYNGEAL GROOVES (1–4) are invaginations of ectoderm located between each pharyngeal arch.

D. PHARYNGEAL MEMBRANES (1–4) are structures consisting of ectoderm, intervening mesoderm and neural crest, and endoderm located between each pharyngeal arch.

II Development of the Thyroid Gland

A. In the midline of the floor of the pharynx, the endodermal lining of the foregut forms the **thyroid diverticulum**.

B. The thyroid diverticulum migrates caudally, passing ventral to the hyoid bone and laryngeal cartilages.

C. During this migration, the thyroid remains connected to the tongue by the **thyroglossal duct**, which is later obliterated.

D. The site of the thyroglossal duct is indicated in the adult by the **foramen cecum**.

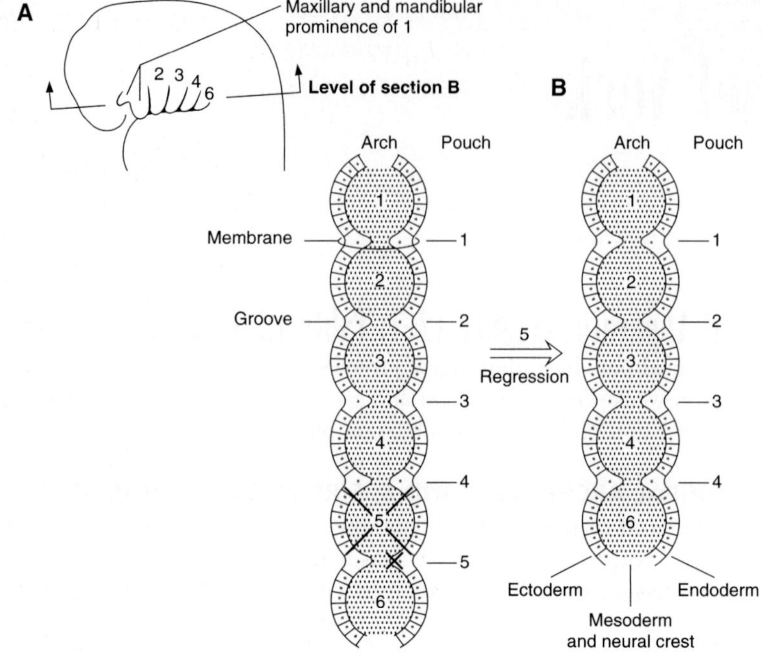

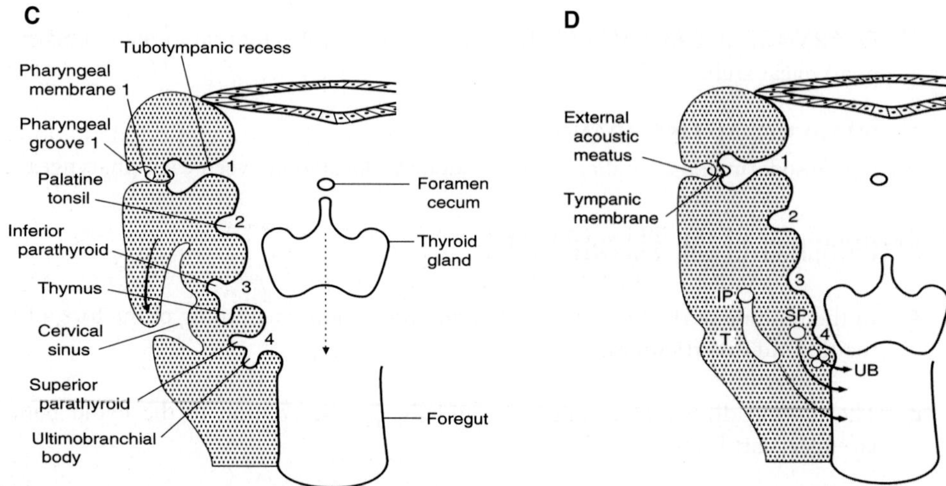

● **Figure 12-1 (A)** Lateral view of an embryo in week 4 of development, showing the pharyngeal arches. Note that pharyngeal arch 1 consists of a maxillary prominence and a mandibular prominence, which can cause some confusion in numbering of the arches. **(B)** A schematic diagram indicating a convenient way to understand the numbering of the arches and pouches. The X's indicate regression of pharyngeal arch 5 and pouch 5. **(C, D)** Schematic diagrams of the fate of the pharyngeal pouches, grooves, and membranes. **(C)** Solid arrow indicates the downward growth of pharyngeal arch 2, thereby forming a smooth contour at the neck region. Dotted arrow indicates downward migration of the thyroid gland. **(D)** Curved arrows indicate the direction of migration of the inferior parathyroid (IP), thymus (T), superior parathyroid (SP), and ultimobranchial bodies (UB). Note that the parathyroid tissue derived from pharyngeal pouch 3 is carried farther caudally by the descent of the thymus than parathyroid tissue from pharyngeal pouch 4.

TABLE 12-1 ADULT DERIVATIVES OF PHARYNGEAL ARCHES, POUCHES, GROOVES, AND MEMBRANES

	Nerve	Adult Derivatives
Arch		
1	CN V	**Mesoderm:** muscles of mastication, mylohyoid, anterior belly of digastric, tensor veli palatini, tensor tympani **Neural crest:** maxilla, mandible, incus, malleus, zygomatic bone, squamous temporal bone, palatine bone, vomer, sphenomandibular ligament
2	CN VII	**Mesoderm:** muscles of facial expression, posterior belly of digastric, stylohyoid, stapedius **Neural crest:** stapes, styloid process, stylohyoid ligament, lesser horn and upper body of hyoid bone
3	CN IX	**Mesoderm:** stylopharyngeus, common carotid arteries, internal carotid arteries **Neural crest:** greater horn and lower body of hyoid bone
4	CN X (superior laryngeal nerve)	**Mesoderm:** muscles of soft palate (except tensor veli palatini), muscles of the pharynx (except stylopharyngeus) cricothyroid, cricopharyngeus, laryngeal cartilages, right subclavian artery, arch of aorta **Neural crest:** none
6	CN X (recurrent laryngeal nerve)	**Mesoderm:** intrinsic muscles of larynx (except cricothyroid), upper muscles of the esophagus, laryngeal cartilages, pulmonary arteries, ductus arteriosus **Neural crest:** none
Pouch		
1		Epithelial lining of auditory tube and middle ear cavity
2		Epithelial lining of palatine tonsil crypts
3		Inferior parathyroid gland, thymus
4		Superior parathyroid gland, ultimobranchial body[a]
Groove		
1		Epithelial lining of the external auditory meatus
2–4		Obliterated
Membrane		
1		Tympanic membrane
2–4		Obliterated

[a]Neural crest cells migrate into the ultimobranchial body to form parafollicular cells (C cells) of the thyroid, which secrete calcitonin.

Development of the Tongue (Figure 12-2)

A. ORAL PART (ANTERIOR 2/3) OF THE TONGUE

1. Forms from the **median tongue bud** and **two distal tongue buds** that develop in the floor of the pharynx associated with **pharyngeal arch 1**.
2. The distal tongue buds overgrow the median tongue bud and fuse in the midline, forming the **median sulcus**.
3. The oral part is characterized by **filiform papillae** (no taste buds), **fungiform papillae** (taste buds present), **foliate papillae** (taste buds present), and **circumvallate papillae** (taste buds present).
4. General sensation from the mucosa is carried by the **lingual branch of the trigeminal nerve (CN V)**.
5. Taste sensation from the mucosa is carried by the **chorda tympani branch of the facial nerve (CN VII)**.

B. PHARYNGEAL PART (POSTERIOR 1/3) OF THE TONGUE

1. Forms from the **copula** and **hypobranchial eminence** that develop in the floor of the pharynx associated with **pharyngeal arches 2–4**.
2. The hypobranchial eminence overgrows the copula, thereby eliminating any contribution of pharyngeal arch 2 in the formation of the definitive adult tongue.
3. The line of fusion between the oral and the pharyngeal parts of the tongue is indicated by the **terminal sulcus**.
4. The pharyngeal part is characterized by the **lingual tonsil**, which forms along with the palatine tonsil and pharyngeal tonsil (adenoids), **Waldeyer's ring**.
5. General sensation from the mucosa is carried primarily by the **glossopharyngeal nerve (CN IX)**.
6. Taste sensation from the mucosa is carried predominantly by the **glossopharyngeal nerve (CN IX)**.

C. MUSCLES OF THE TONGUE

1. The intrinsic muscles and extrinsic muscles (styloglossus, hyoglossus, genioglossus, and palatoglossus) are derived from myoblasts that migrate into the tongue region from **occipital somites**.
2. Motor innervation is supplied by the **hypoglossal nerve (CN XII)**, except for the palatoglossus muscle, which is innervated by CN X.

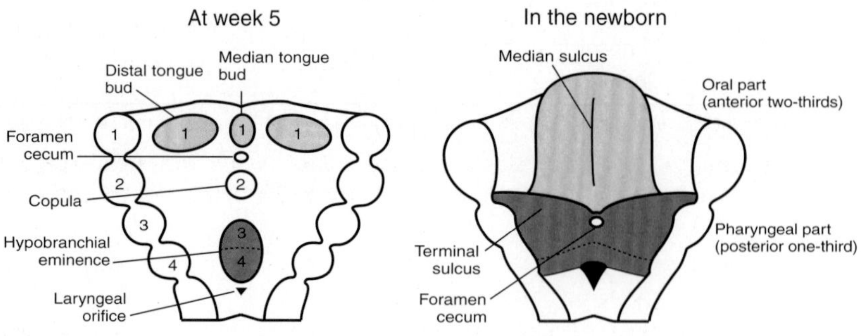

Figure 12-2 Development of the tongue at week 5 and in the newborn.

IV Development of the Face (Figure 12-3)

A. The face is formed by three swellings: the **frontonasal prominence**, the **maxillary prominence** (pharyngeal arch 1), and the **mandibular prominence** (pharyngeal arch 1).

B. Bilateral ectodermal thickenings called **nasal placodes** develop on the ventrolateral aspects of the frontonasal prominence.

C. The nasal placodes invaginate into the underlying mesoderm to form the **nasal pits**, thereby producing a ridge of tissue that forms the **medial nasal prominence** and **the lateral nasal prominence**.

D. A deep groove called the **nasolacrimal groove** forms between the maxillary prominence and the lateral nasal prominence and eventually forms the **nasolacrimal duct** and **lacrimal sac**.

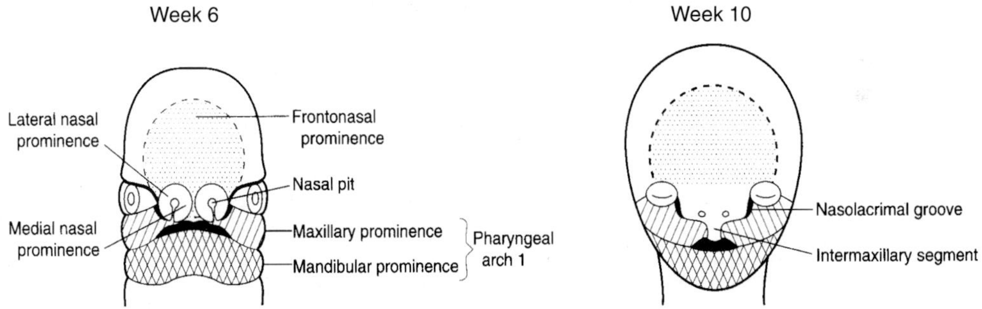

● **Figure 12-3** Development of the face at week 6 and week 10.

V Development of the Palate (Figure 12-4)

A. INTERMAXILLARY SEGMENT

1. Forms when the medial growth of the maxillary prominences causes the two medial nasal prominences to fuse together at the midline.
2. The intermaxillary segment forms the **philtrum of the lip**, **four incisor teeth**, and **primary palate**.

B. SECONDARY PALATE

1. Forms from outgrowths of the maxillary prominences called the **palatine shelves**.
2. Initially the palatine shelves project downward on either side of the tongue but later attain a horizontal position and fuse along the **palatine raphe** to form the **secondary palate**.
3. The primary and secondary palate fuse at the **incisive foramen** to form the **definitive palate**. Bone develops in both the primary palate and the anterior part of the secondary palate.
4. Bone does not develop in the posterior part of the secondary palate, which eventually forms the **soft palate** and **uvula**.
5. The **nasal septum** develops from the medial nasal prominences and fuses with the definitive palate.

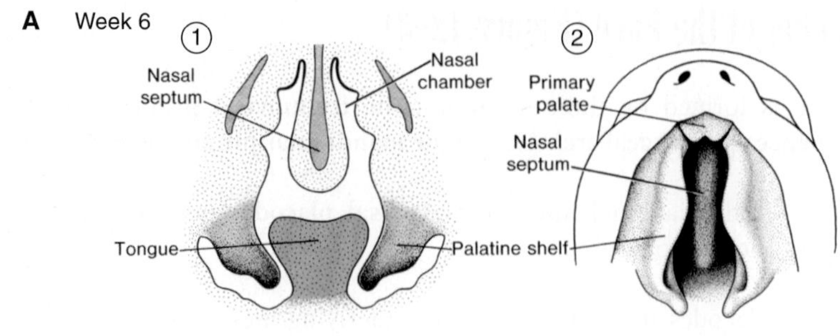

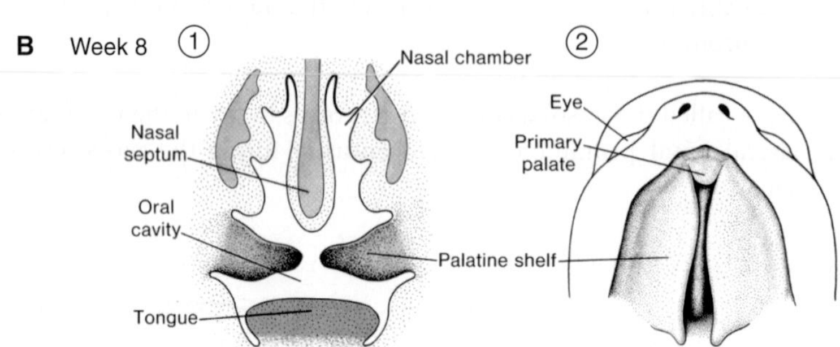

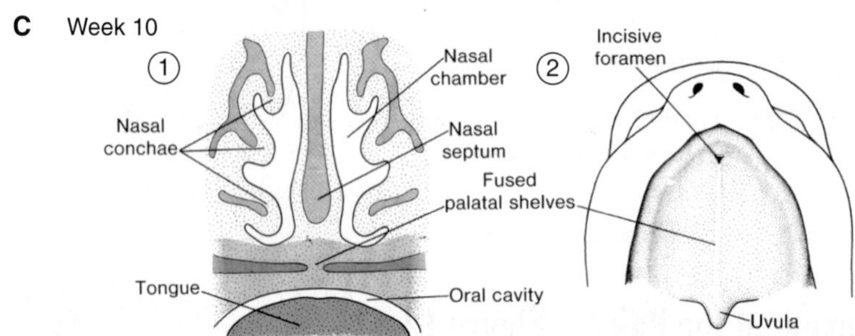

● **Figure 12-4** Development of the palate at week 6, week 8, and week 10. (1) Horizontal sections (2) Roof of the mouth.

VI Clinical Considerations

A. FIRST ARCH SYNDROME (FIGURE 12-5) results from abnormal development of **pharyngeal arch 1** and produces various facial anomalies. It is caused by a lack of migration of neural crest cells into pharyngeal arch 1. Two well-described first arch syndromes are **Treacher Collins syndrome (mandibulofacial dysostosis)** and **Pierre Robin syndrome.** Figure 12-5 shows Treacher Collins syndrome (mandibulofacial dysostosis), which is characterized by underdevelopment of the zygomatic bones, mandibular hypoplasia, lower eyelid colobomas, downward-slanting palpebral fissures, and malformed external ears (note the hearing aid cord). Treacher Collins

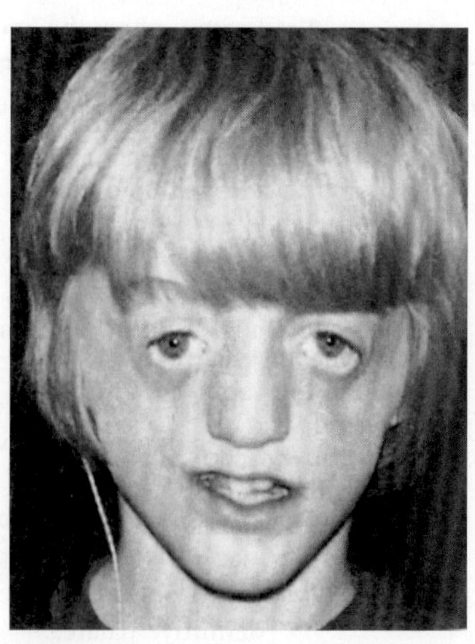

● **Figure 12-5 Treacher Collins syndrome (Mandibulofacial Dysostosis).**

syndrome is an autosomal dominant genetic disorder caused by a mutation in the TCOF1 gene on chromosome 5q32.3-q33.1 for the **treacle protein**.

B. PHARYNGEAL FISTULA (FIGURE 12-6) occurs when **pharyngeal pouch** 2 and **pharyngeal groove 2** persist, thereby forming a patent opening from the internal tonsillar area to the external neck. It is generally found along the **anterior border of the sternocleidomastoid muscle.** The computed tomography (CT) scan in Figure 12-6 shows a low-density mass (B) just anteromedial to the sternocleidomastoid muscle (M) and anterolateral to the carotid artery and jugular vein (arrows). The pharyngeal cyst arises from a persistence of pharyngeal groove 2. This may also involve the persistence of pharyngeal pouch 2, thereby forming a patent opening of fistula through the neck. The fistula may begin inside the throat near the tonsils, travel through the neck, and open to the outside near the anterior border of the sternocleidomastoid muscle.

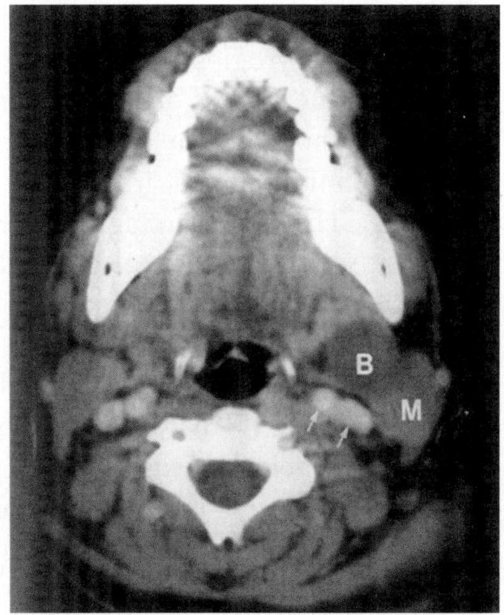

● **Figure 12-6 Pharyngeal cyst/fistula.**

C. PHARYNGEAL CYST (FIGURE 12-7) occurs when parts of the **pharyngeal grooves 2–4** that are normally obliterated persist, thereby forming a cyst. It is generally found near the **angle of the mandible**. Figure 12-7 shows a fluid-filled cyst (circle) near the angle of the mandible (*arrow*).

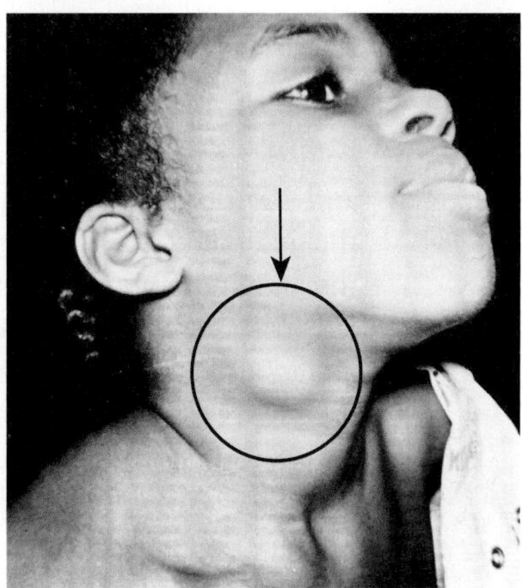

● **Figure 12-7 Pharyngeal cyst.**

D. ECTOPIC THYMUS, PARATHYROID, OR THYROID TISSUE (FIGURE 12-8) result from the abnormal migration of these glands from their embryonic position to their definitive adult location. Glandular tissue may be found anywhere along their migratory path. Figure 12-8 shows **ectopic thyroid tissue.** A sublingual thyroid mass (arrow) is seen in this young euthyroid child.

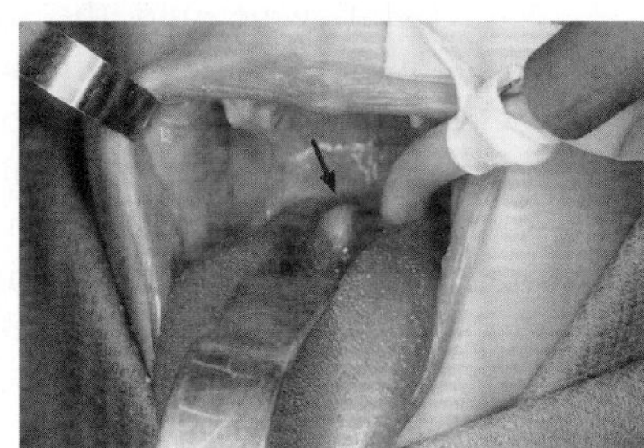

● **Figure 12-8 Ectopic thyroid tissue.**

E. THYROGLOSSAL DUCT CYST (FIGURE 12-9) occurs when parts of the thyroglossal duct persist and thereby form a cyst. It is most commonly located in the midline near the hyoid bone, but it may also be located at the base of the tongue, in which case it is then called a **lingual**

cyst. The top photograph in Figure 12-9 shows a thyroglossal duct cyst (*arrow*). A thyroglossal duct cyst is one of the most frequent congenital anomalies in the neck and is found along the midline most frequently below the hyoid bone. The bottom magnetic resonance image (MRI) shows a mass of thyroid tissue (*arrow*) at the base of the tongue called a lingual cyst.

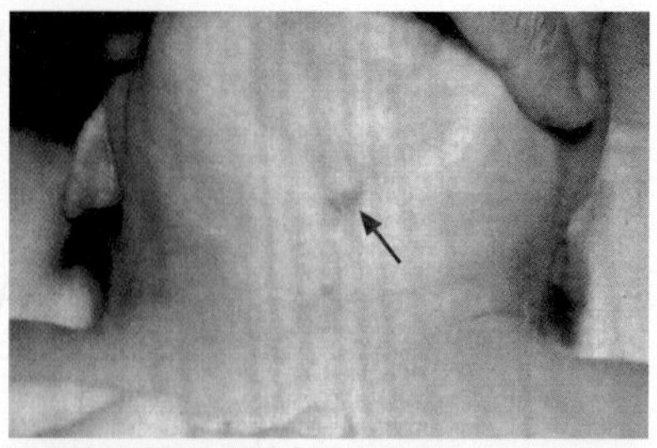

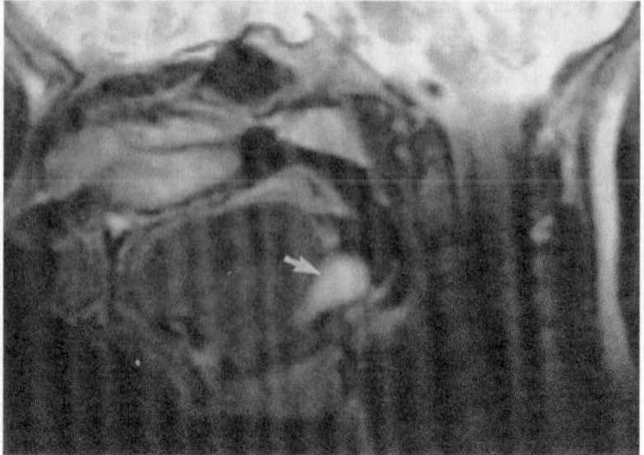

● **Figure 12-9 Thyroglossal duct cyst/ Lingual cyst.**

F. **CONGENITAL HYPOTHYROIDISM (CRETINISM) (FIGURE 12-10)** occurs when a thyroid deficiency exists during the early fetal period due to a severe lack of dietary iodine, thyroid agenesis, or mutations involving the biosynthesis of thyroid hormone. This condition causes impaired skeletal growth and mental retardation. This condition is characterized by coarse facial features, a low-set hair line, sparse eyebrows, wide-set eyes, periorbital puffiness, a flat, broad nose, an enlarged, protuberant tongue, a hoarse cry, umbilical hernia, dry and cold extremities, dry, rough skin (myxedema), and mottled skin. It is important to note that the majority of infants with congenital hypothyroidism have no physical stigmata. This has led to screening of all newborns in the United States and in most other developed countries for depressed thyroxin or elevated thyroid-stimulating hormone levels. Figure 12-10 shows an infant with congenital hypothyroidism.

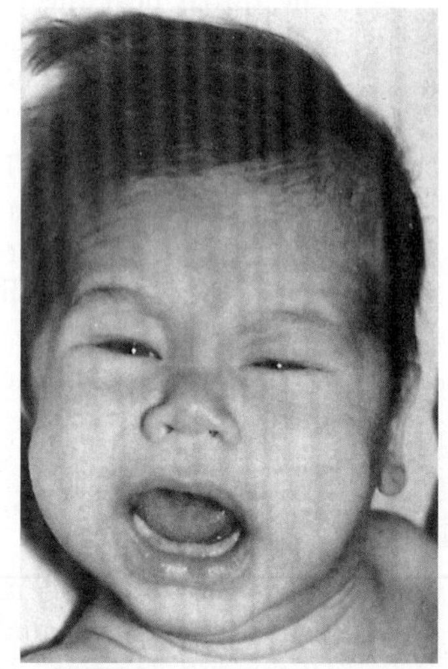

● **Figure 12-10 Congenital hypothyroidism (cretinism).**

G. **OROFACIAL CLEFTING (FIGURE 12-11)** is a multifactorial genetic disorder involving the *DLX* gene family, *SHH* gene, *TGF-α* gene, *TGF-ß* gene, and the *IRF-6* gene along with some putative environmental factors (e.g., phenytoin, sodium valproate, methotrexate). The most common craniofacial birth defect is the orofacial cleft, which consists of a **cleft lip with or without cleft palate** (CL/P) or an **isolated cleft palate** (CP). CL/P and CP are distinct birth defects (even though they often occur together) based on their embryological formation, etiology, candidate genes, and recurrence risk. Figure 12-11 shows a young child with a unilateral cleft lip with a cleft palate (CL/P).

1. **Cleft lip** is a multifactorial genetic disorder that involves neural crest cells. Cleft lip results from the following:
   - The maxillary prominence fails to fuse with the medial nasal prominence.

- The underlying mesoderm and neural crest fail to expand, resulting in a **persistent labial groove**.

2. **Cleft palate** is a multifactorial genetic disorder that involves neural crest cells. Cleft palate is classified as anterior or posterior. The anatomic landmark that distinguishes an anterior cleft palate from a posterior cleft palate is the **incisive foramen**.
   a. **Anterior cleft palate**
      - Occurs when the palatine shelves fail to fuse with the primary palate.
   b. **Posterior cleft palate**
      - Occurs when the palatine shelves fail to fuse with each other and with the nasal septum.
   c. **Anteroposterior cleft palate**
      - Occurs when there is a combination of both defects.

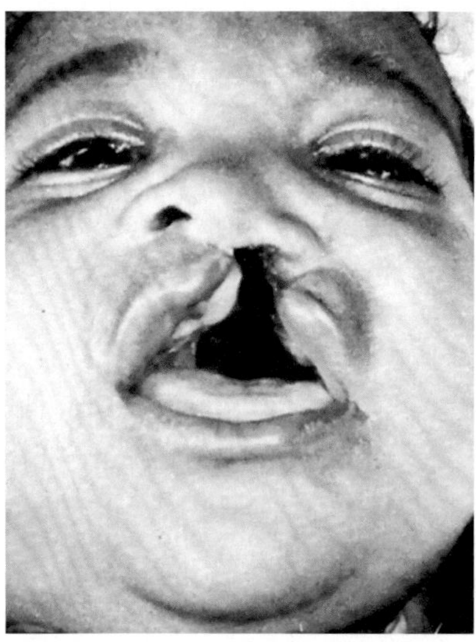

● **Figure 12-11 Unilateral cleft lip with a cleft palate (CL/P).**

H. **DIGEORGE SYNDROME (DS)** occurs when **pharyngeal pouches 3 and 4** fail to differentiate into the thymus and parathyroid glands. DS is usually accompanied by facial anomalies resembling first arch syndrome (micrognathia, low-set ears) due to abnormal neural crest cell migration, cardiovascular anomalies due to abnormal neural crest cell migration during formation of the aorticopulmonary septum, immunodeficiency due to absence of thymus gland, and hypocalcemia due to absence of parathyroid glands.

Case Study

While delivering a newborn baby girl you notice that she has abnormal facies, as well as a cleft palate. What is the most likely diagnosis?

Differentials

- First arch syndrome, DS

Relevant Physical Exam Findings

- No detectable thymus on palpation
- Cleft palate
- Muscle rigidity

Relevant Lab Findings

- Hypocalcemia
- X-ray congenital heart disease
- Genetic testing shows a 22q deletion.

Diagnosis

- **DS:** A first arch syndrome shows abnormal facies and cleft palate. However, DS presents with those conditions as well as with hypocalcemia, 22q deletion, and tetany.

Chapter **13**

Nervous System

I Development of the Neural Tube (Figure 13-1).

Neurulation refers to the formation and closure of the neural tube. The events of neurulation occur as follows:

A. The **notochord** induces the overlying ectoderm to differentiate into **neuroectoderm** and form the **neural plate**. The notochord forms the **nucleus pulposus** of the intervertebral disk in the adult.

B. The neural plate folds to give rise to the **neural tube**, which is open at both ends at the **anterior** and **posterior neuropores**. The anterior and posterior neuropores connect the lumen of the neural tube with the amniotic cavity.

C. The **anterior neuropore** closes during week 4 (day 25) and becomes the **lamina terminalis**. Failure of the anterior neuropore to close results in upper neural tube defects (NTDs; e.g., **anencephaly**).

D. The **posterior neuropore** closes during week 4 (day 27). Failure of the posterior neuropore to close results in lower NTDs (e.g., **spina bifida with myeloschisis**).

E. As the neural plate folds, some cells differentiate into **neural crest cells** and form a column of cells along both sides of the neural tube.

F. The rostral part of the neural tube becomes the **adult brain**.

G. The caudal part of the neural tube becomes the **adult spinal cord**.

H. The lumen of the neural tube gives rise to the **ventricular system** of the brain and **central canal** of the spinal cord.

II Neural Crest Cells.

The neural crest cells differentiate from neuroectoderm of the neural tube and form a column of cells along both sides of the neural tube. Neural crest cells undergo a prolific migration throughout the embryo (both the cranial region and the trunk region) and ultimately differentiate into a wide array of adult cells and structures, as indicated in the following.

A. CRANIAL REGION NEURAL CREST CELLS. Cranial region neural crest cells differentiate into the following adult cells and structures: **pharyngeal arch skeletal and connective tissue components; bones of neurocranium; pia and arachnoid; parafollicular (C) cells of thyroid; aorticopulmonary septum; odontoblasts (dentin of teeth); sensory ganglia of CN V, CN VII, CN IX, and CN X; ciliary (CN III), pterygopalatine (CN VII), submandibular (CN VII), and otic (CN IX) parasympathetic ganglia.**

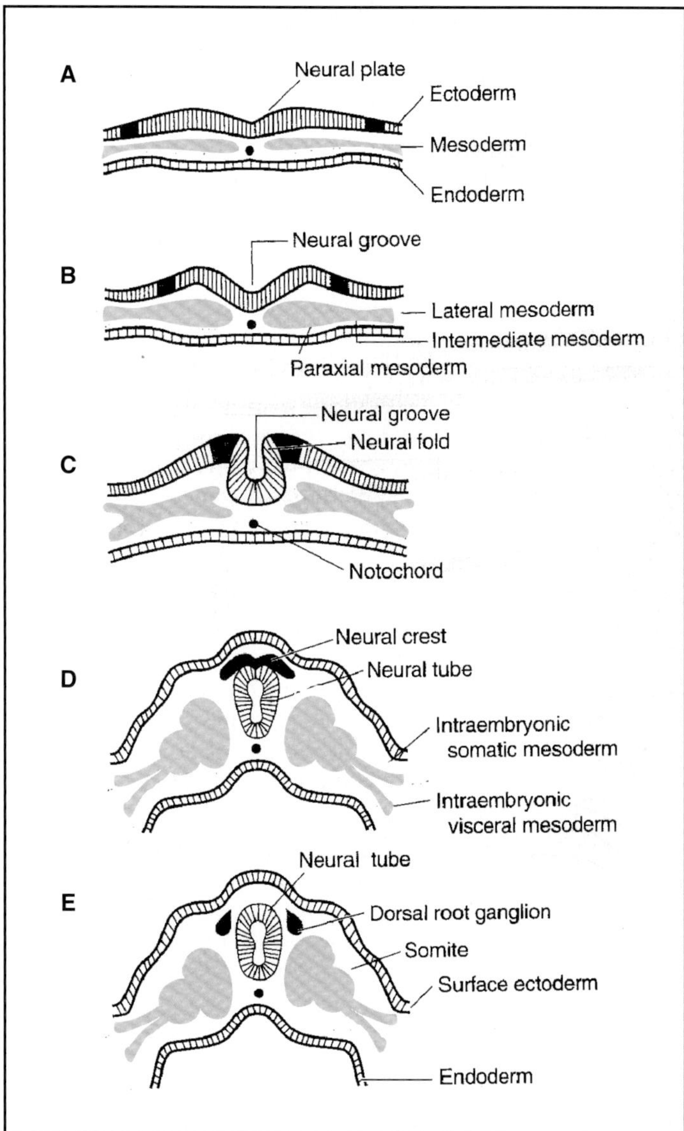

● **Figure 13-1 Schematic diagrams of transverse sections of embryos at various stages. (A)** Neural plate stage. **(B)** Early neural groove stage. **(C)** Late neural groove stage. **(D)** Early neural tube and neural crest stage. **(E)** Neural tube and dorsal root ganglion stage.

B. TRUNK REGION NEURAL CREST CELLS. Trunk region neural crest cells differentiate into the following adult cells and structures: **melanocytes, Schwann cells, chromaffin cells of adrenal medulla, dorsal root ganglia, sympathetic chain ganglia, prevertebral sympathetic ganglia, enteric parasympathetic ganglia of the gut (Meissner and Auerbach; CN X), and abdominal/pelvic cavity parasympathetic ganglia.**

C. CLINICAL CONSIDERATIONS. Neurocristopathy is a term used to describe any disease related to maldevelopment of neural crest cells. Some neurocristopathies are indicated in the following.

1. **Medullary carcinoma (MC) of thyroid.** MC of thyroid is an endocrine neoplasm of the par afollicular (C) cells of neural crest origin that secrete calcitonin. The

carcinoma cells are usually arranged in cell nests surrounded by bands of stroma containing amyloid.

2. **Schwannoma.** A schwannoma is a benign tumor of Schwann cells of neural crest origin. These tumors are well-circumscribed, encapsulated masses that may or may not be attached to the nerve. The most common location within the cranial vault is at the cerebellopontine angle near the vestibular branch of CN VIII (often referred to as an **acoustic neuroma**). Clinical findings include tinnitus and hearing loss. CN V (trigeminal nerve) is also commonly affected.
3. **Neurofibromatosis type 1 (NF1; von Recklinghausen disease).** NF1 is a relatively common autosomal dominant disorder caused by a mutation in the **NF1 gene** on chromosome 17q11.2 for the protein **neurofibromin**. Neurofibromin downregulates **p21 ras oncoprotein** so that the NF1 gene belongs to the family of tumor-suppressor genes. Clinical findings include multiple neural tumors (called **neurofibromas**), which are widely dispersed over the body and reveal proliferation of all elements of a peripheral nerve, including neurites, fibroblasts, and Schwann cells of neural crest origin, numerous pigmented skin lesions (called **café au lait spots**), probably associated with melanocytes of neural crest origin, and pigmented iris hamartomas (called **Lisch nodules**).
4. **CHARGE association.** The CHARGE association is understandable only if the wide distribution of neural crest cell derivatives is appreciated. The cause of the CHARGE is unknown but seems to involve an insult during the second month of gestation probably involving the neural crest cells. Clinical findings include **c**oloboma of the retina, lens, or choroid; **h**eart defects (e.g., tetralogy of Fallot, ventricular septal defect [VSD], patent ductus arteriosus [PDA]); **a**tresia choanae; **r**etardation of growth; **g**enital abnormalities in male infants (e.g., cryptorchidism, microphallus); and **e**ar abnormalities or deafness.
5. **Waardenburg syndrome (WS).** WS is an autosomal dominant disorder caused by a mutation in either the ***PAX3* gene** on chromosome 2q35 (Type I WS) for a **paired box *PAX3* transcription factor** or the **MITF gene** on chromosome 3p12.3-p12.3 (Type II WS) for the microphthalmia-associated transcription factor. Clinical findings include malposition of the eyelid, lateral displacement of lacrimal puncta, a broad nasal root, heterochromia of the iris, congenital deafness, and piebaldism, including a white forelock and a triangular area of hypopigmentation.

III Vesicle Development of the Neural Tube (Figure 13-2)

A. PRIMARY BRAIN VESICLES. The three **primary brain vesicles** and two associated **flexures** develop during week 4.

1. **Prosencephalon (forebrain)** gives rise to the **telencephalon** and **diencephalons**.
2. **Mesencephalon (midbrain)** remains as the **mesencephalon**.
3. **Rhombencephalon (hindbrain)** gives rise to the **metencephalon** and the **myelencephalon**.
4. **Cephalic flexure (midbrain flexure)** is located between the **prosencephalon** and the **rhombencephalon**.
5. **Cervical flexure** is located between the rhombencephalon and the future spinal cord.

B. SECONDARY BRAIN VESICLES. The five **secondary brain vesicles** develop during week 6 and form various adult derivatives of the brain.

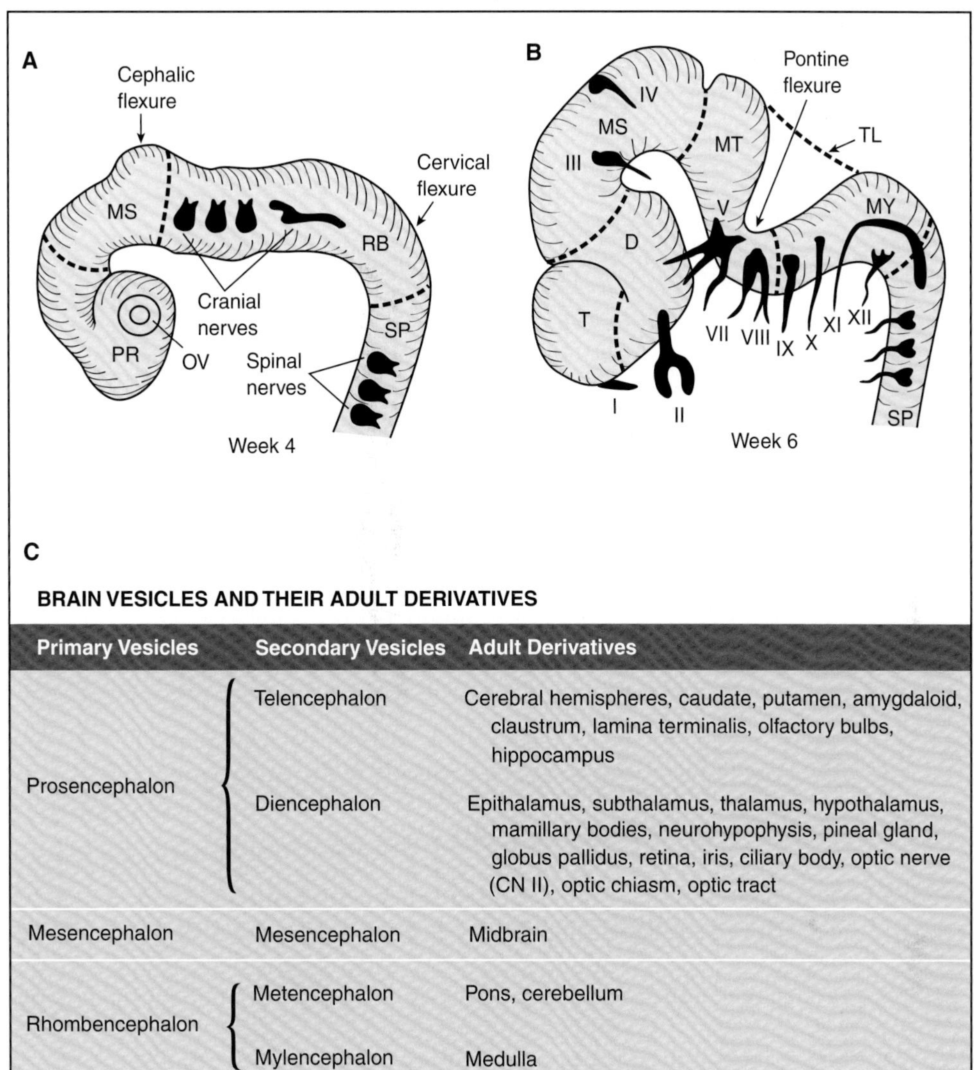

BRAIN VESICLES AND THEIR ADULT DERIVATIVES

Primary Vesicles	Secondary Vesicles	Adult Derivatives
Prosencephalon	Telencephalon	Cerebral hemispheres, caudate, putamen, amygdaloid, claustrum, lamina terminalis, olfactory bulbs, hippocampus
	Diencephalon	Epithalamus, subthalamus, thalamus, hypothalamus, mamillary bodies, neurohypophysis, pineal gland, globus pallidus, retina, iris, ciliary body, optic nerve (CN II), optic chiasm, optic tract
Mesencephalon	Mesencephalon	Midbrain
Rhombencephalon	Metencephalon	Pons, cerebellum
	Mylencephalon	Medulla

● **Figure 13-2 Schematic illustrations of the developing brain vesicles. (A)** Three-vesicle stage of the brain in a 4-week-old embryo. Divisions are indicated by dashed lines. MS = mesencephalon; OV = optic vesicle; PR = prosencephalon; RB = rhombencephalon; SP = spinal cord. **(B)** Five-vesicle stage of the brain in a 6-week-old embryo. Divisions are indicated by dashed lines. Cranial nerves (CN) are indicated by Roman numerals. CN VI is not shown because it exits the brainstem from the ventral surface. D = diencephalons; MS = mesencephalon; MT = metencephalon; MY = myelencephalon; SP = spinal cord; T = telencephalon; TL = tela choroidea. **(C)** Table indicating the brain vesicles and their adult derivatives.

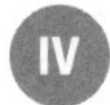 Development of the Spinal Cord.

The spinal cord develops from the neural tube.

A. THE ALAR (SENSORY) PLATE

1. Is a **dorsolateral** thickening of the intermediate zone of the neural tube.
2. Gives rise to **sensory neuroblasts of the dorsal horn.**
3. Receives axons from the dorsal root ganglia, which enter the spinal cord and become the **dorsal (sensory) roots.**
4. The alar plate eventually becomes the **dorsal horn of the spinal cord.**

B. THE BASAL (MOTOR) PLATE

1. Is a **ventrolateral** thickening of the intermediate zone of the neural tube.
2. Gives rise to **motor neuroblasts of the ventral and lateral horns.**
3. Projects axons from motor neuroblasts, which exit the spinal cord and become the **ventral (motor) roots.**
4. The basal plate eventually becomes the **ventral horn of the spinal cord.**

C. SULCUS LIMITANS

1. Is a **longitudinal groove** in the lateral wall of the neural tube that appears during week 4 of development and separates the alar and basal plates.
2. Extends from the spinal cord to the rostral midbrain.

D. CAUDAL EMINENCE

1. Arises from the primitive streak and blends with the neural tube.
2. Gives rise to **sacral and coccygeal segments of the spinal cord.**

E. MYELINATION OF THE SPINAL CORD

1. Begins during month 4 in the ventral (motor) roots.
2. **Oligodendrocytes** accomplish myelination in the **central nervous system** (CNS), and **Schwann cells** accomplish myelination in the **peripheral nervous system** (PNS).
3. Myelination of the **corticospinal tracts** is not completed until the end of 2 years of age.
4. Myelination of the **association neocortex** extends to 30 years of age.

F. POSITIONAL CHANGES OF THE SPINAL CORD (FIGURE 13-3)

1. **At week 8** of development, the spinal cord extends the length of the vertebral canal.
2. **At birth,** the **conus medullaris** extends to the level of the third lumbar vertebra (L3).
3. **In adults,** the conus medullaris terminates at **L1–L2 interspace.**
4. Disparate growth (between the vertebral column and the spinal cord) results in the formation of the **cauda equina**, consisting of dorsal and ventral roots, which descends below the level of the conus medullaris.
5. Disparate growth results in the nonneural **filum terminale**, which anchors the spinal cord to the coccyx.

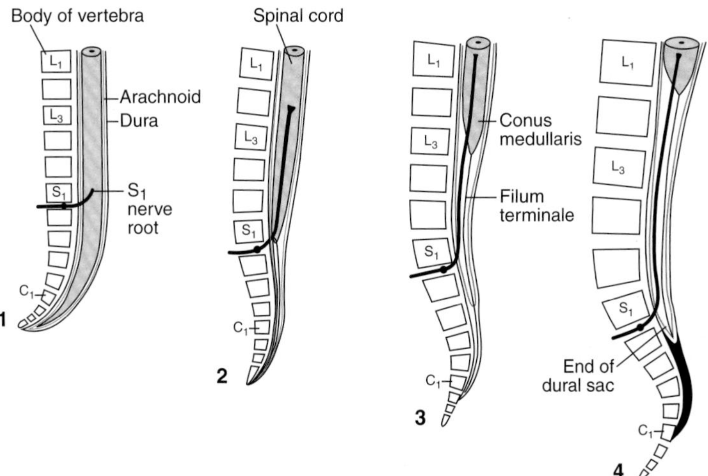

● **Figure 13-3 Positional changes in the spinal cord.** The end of the spinal cord (conus medullaris) is shown in relation to the vertebral column and meninges. **(1)** Week 8, **(2)** week 24, **(3)** newborn, **(4)** adult. As the vertebral column grows, nerve roots (especially those of the lumbar and sacral segments) are elongated to form the cauda equina. The S1 nerve root is shown as an example.

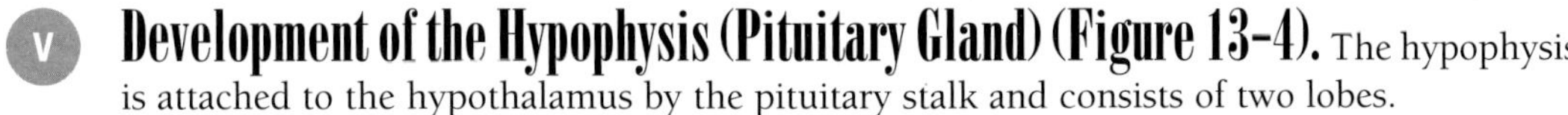

V Development of the Hypophysis (Pituitary Gland) (Figure 13-4).

The hypophysis is attached to the hypothalamus by the pituitary stalk and consists of two lobes.

A. ANTERIOR LOBE (ADENOHYPOPHYSIS), PARS TUBERALIS, AND PARS INTERMEDIA

1. Develop from **Rathke's pouch**, which is an ectodermal diverticulum of the primitive mouth cavity (stomodeum).
2. Remnants of Rathke's pouch may give rise to a **craniopharyngioma.**

B. POSTERIOR LOBE (NEUROHYPOPHYSIS) develops from the **infundibulum**, which is a neuroectodermal diverticulum of the hypothalamus.

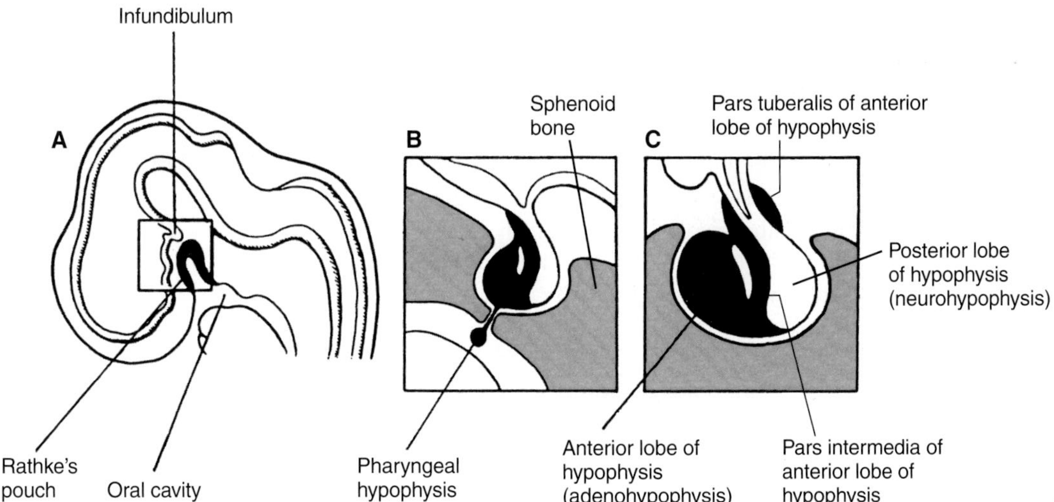

● **Figure 13-4 Development of the hypophysis. (A)** A midsagittal section through a week 6 embryo showing Rathke's pouch as a dorsal outpocketing of the oral cavity and the infundibulum as a thickening in the floor of the hypothalamus. **(B, C)** Development at weeks 11 and 16, respectively. The anterior lobe, pars tuberalis, and pars intermedia are derived from Rathke's pouch.

VI Congenital Malformations of the Central Nervous System

A. VARIATIONS OF SPINA BIFIDA (FIGURE 13-5). Spina bifida occurs when the **bony vertebral arches** fail to form properly, thereby creating a vertebral defect usually in the **lumbosacral region.** It is due primarily to expectant mothers not taking enough **folic acid** during pregnancy.

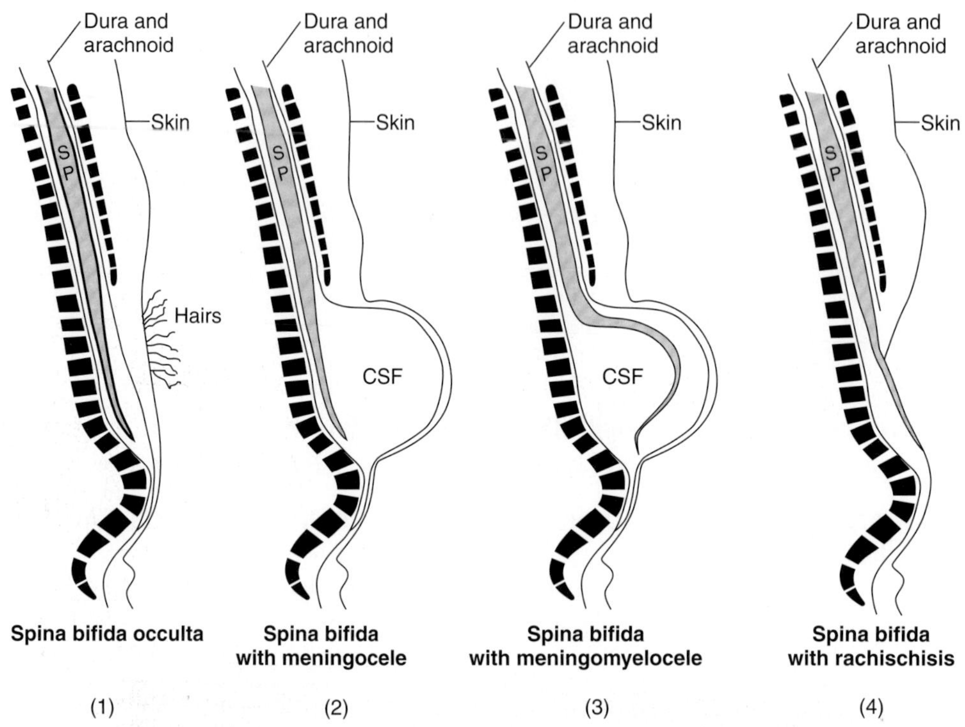

● **Figure 13-5 Schematic drawings illustrating the various types of spina bifida. (1)** Spina bifida occulta, **(2)** spina bifida with meningocele, **(3)** spina bifida with meningomyelocele, **(4)** spina bifida with rachischisis. CSF = cerebrospinal fluid.

1. **Spina bifida occulta (Figure 13-6)** is evidenced by multiple dimples present on the back of the infant, which may or may not be accompanied by a tuft of hair in the lumbosacral region. It is the least severe variation and occurs in 10% of the population. In spina bifida occulta the bony vertebral bodies are present along the entire length of the vertebral column. However, the bony spinous processes terminate at a much higher level because the vertebral arches fail to form properly. This creates a bony vertebral defect. The

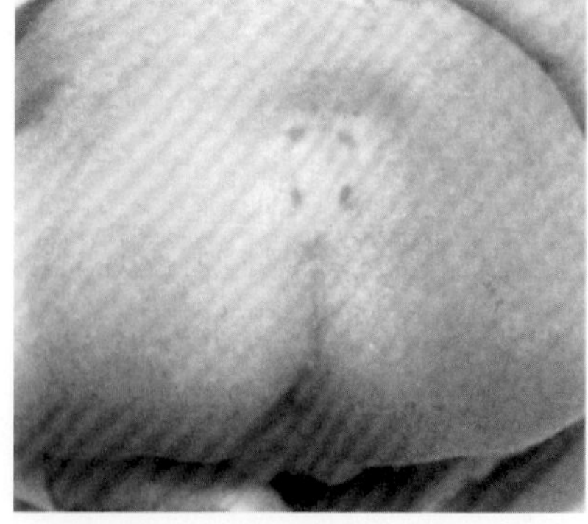

● **Figure 13-6 Spina bifida occulta.**

spinal cord is intact. Figure 13-6 shows the multiple dimples present on the back of an affected infant in the lumbosacral region.

2. **Spina bifida with meningocele** occurs when the meninges protrude through a vertebral defect and form a sac filled with cerebrospinal fluid (CSF). The spinal cord remains in its normal position.
3. **Spina bifida with meningomyelocele** occurs when the meninges and spinal cord protrude through a vertebral defect and form a sac filled with CSF.
4. **Spina bifida with rachischisis (Figure 13-7)** occurs when the posterior neuropore of the neural tube fails to close during week 4 of development. This condition is the most severe type of spina bifida and causes paralysis from the level of the defect caudally. This variation presents clinically as an **open neural tube** that lies on the surface of the back. This condition also falls into a classification called **NTDs**. **Lower NTDs** (i.e., spina bifida with rachischisis) result from a failure of the **posterior neuropore** to close during week 4 of development and usually occur in the lumbosacral region. **Upper NTDs** (e.g., anencephaly) result from a failure of the **anterior neuropore** to close during week 4 of development. NTDs can be diagnosed prenatally by detecting elevated levels of **α-fetoprotein** in the amniotic fluid. About 75% of all NTDs can be prevented if all women capable of becoming pregnant consume **folic acid** (dose: 0.4 mg of folic acid/day). Figure 13-7 shows an affected newborn infant with the open neural tube on the back.

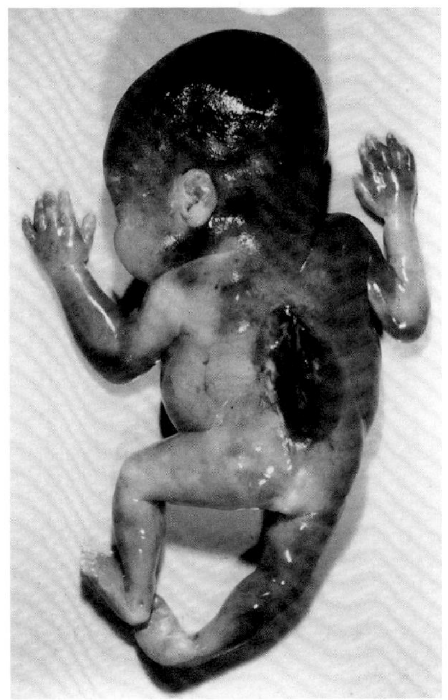

● Figure 13-7 Spina bifida with rachischisis.

B. VARIATIONS OF CRANIUM BIFIDA (FIGURE 13-8). Cranium bifida occurs when the **bony skull** fails to form properly, thereby creating a skull defect usually in the **occipital region.** It is due primarily to expectant mothers not taking enough **folic acid** during pregnancy.

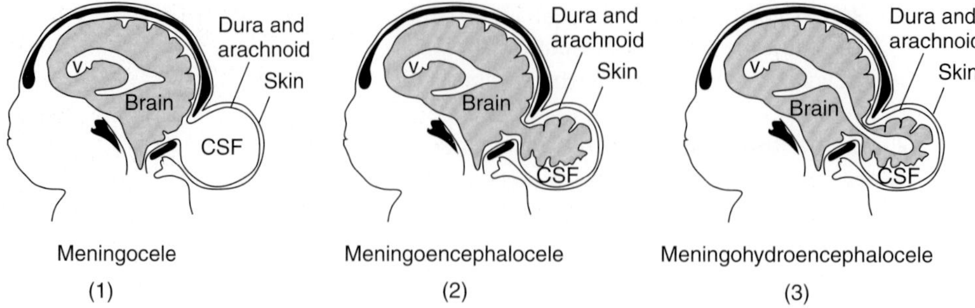

● **Figure 13-8 Schematic drawings illustrating the various types of cranium bifidum. (1)** Cranium bifida with meningocele, **(2)** cranium bifida with meningoencephalocele, **(3)** cranium bifida with meningohydroencephalocele. CSF, cerebrospinal fluid.

1. **Cranium bifida with meningocele (Figure 13-9)** occurs when the meninges protrude through the skull defect and form a sac filled with CSF. Figure 13-9 shows an infant with an occipital meningocele.
2. **Cranium bifida with meningoencephalocele (Figure 13-10)** occurs when the meninges and brain protrude through the skull defect and form a sac filled with CSF. This defect usually comes to medical attention within the infant's first few days or weeks of life. The outcome is poor (i.e., 75% of the infants die or have severe retardation). The magnetic resonance image (MRI) in Figure 13-10 shows a large meningoencephalocele (arrows) extending through an occipital bone defect that contains meninges and brain tissue (B).
3. **Cranium bifida with meningohydroencephalocele** occurs when the meninges, brain, and a portion of the ventricle protrude through the skull defect.

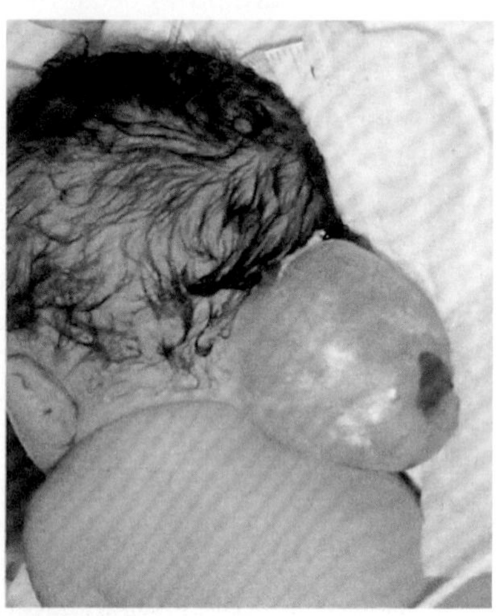

● **Figure 13-9 Cranium bifida with meningocele.**

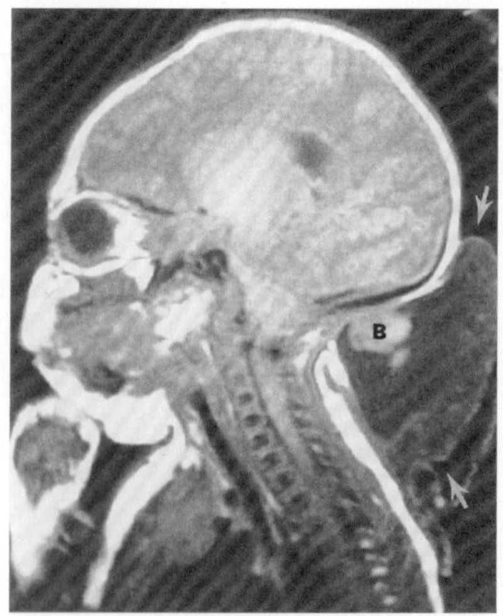

● **Figure 13-10 Cranium bifida with meningoencephalocele.**

C. ANENCEPHALY (MEROANENCEPHALY). Anencephaly is a type of **upper NTD** that occurs when the **anterior neuropore** fails to close during week 4 (day 25) of development. This results in failure of the brain to develop (however, a rudimentary brain is present), failure of the lamina terminalis to form, and failure of the bony cranial vault to form. Anencephaly is incompatible with extrauterine life. If not stillborn, infants with anencephaly survive from only a few hours to a few weeks. Anencephaly is the common serious birth defect seen in stillborn fetuses. Anencephaly is easily diagnosed by ultrasound, and a therapeutic abortion is usually performed at the mother's request. Figure 13-11 shows a newborn infant with anencephaly.

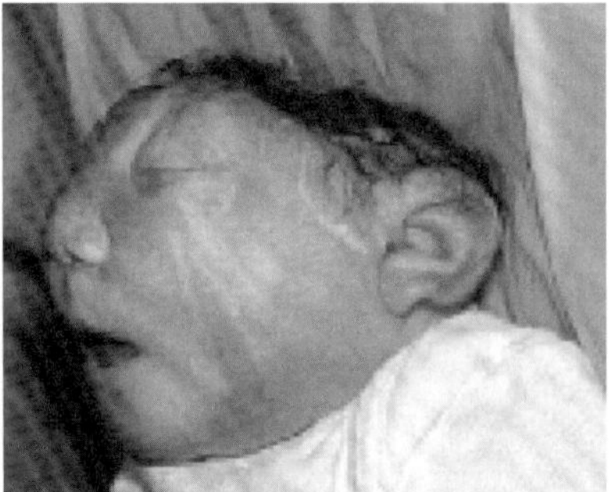

● **Figure 13-11 Anencephaly.**

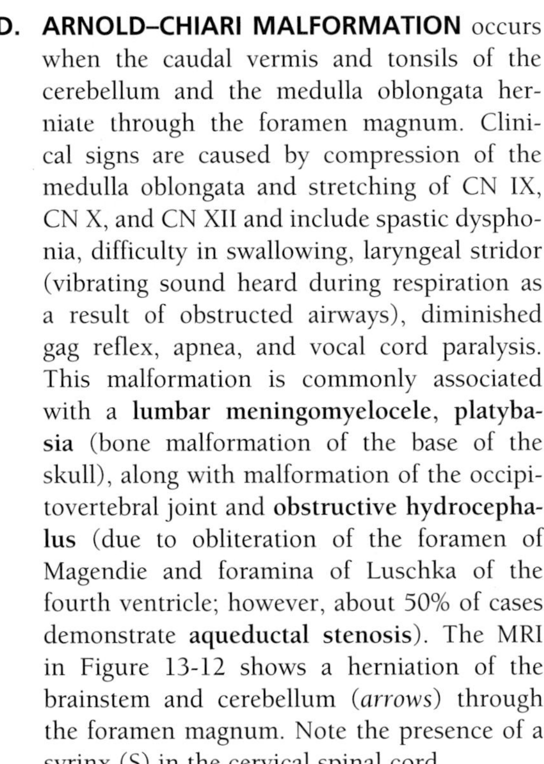

D. ARNOLD–CHIARI MALFORMATION occurs when the caudal vermis and tonsils of the cerebellum and the medulla oblongata herniate through the foramen magnum. Clinical signs are caused by compression of the medulla oblongata and stretching of CN IX, CN X, and CN XII and include spastic dysphonia, difficulty in swallowing, laryngeal stridor (vibrating sound heard during respiration as a result of obstructed airways), diminished gag reflex, apnea, and vocal cord paralysis. This malformation is commonly associated with a **lumbar meningomyelocele, platybasia** (bone malformation of the base of the skull), along with malformation of the occipitovertebral joint and **obstructive hydrocephalus** (due to obliteration of the foramen of Magendie and foramina of Luschka of the fourth ventricle; however, about 50% of cases demonstrate **aqueductal stenosis**). The MRI in Figure 13-12 shows a herniation of the brainstem and cerebellum (*arrows*) through the foramen magnum. Note the presence of a syrinx (S) in the cervical spinal cord.

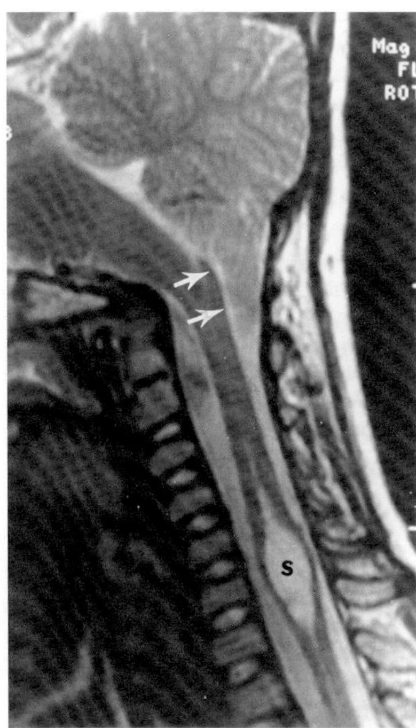

● **Figure 13-12 Arnold–Chiari malformation.**

E. DANDY–WALKER SYNDROME is a type of noncommunicating (or obstructive) hydrocephalus. It is associated with **atresia of the foramen of Magendie and foramina of Luschka** (although it remains controversial). This syndrome is usually associated with dilation of the fourth ventricle, posterior fossa cyst, agenesis of the cerebellar vermis, small cerebellar hemispheres, occipital meningocele, and frequently agenesis of the splenium of the corpus callosum. The MRI in Figure 13-13 shows a dilated fourth ventricle (4) communicating with a posterior fossa cyst (CY) along with small cerebellar hemispheres.

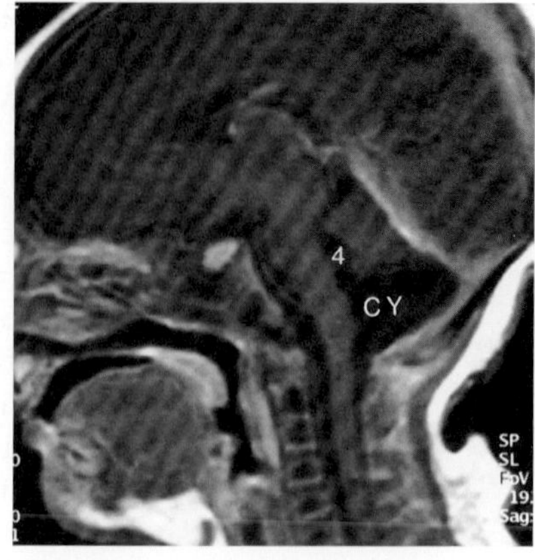

● **Figure 13-13 Dandy–Walker syndrome.** 4 = fourth ventricle; CY = posterior fossa cyst.

F. TETHERED SPINAL CORD (FILUM TERMINALE SYNDROME) occurs when a thick, short filum terminale forms. The result is weakness and sensory deficits in the lower extremity and a neurogenic bladder. A tethered spinal cord is frequently associated with lipomatous tumors or meningomyeloceles. Deficits usually improve after transection. The MRI in Figure 13-14 shows a low-positioned spinal cord (arrows) attached to an intraspinal lipoma (L) typical of a tethered spinal cord.

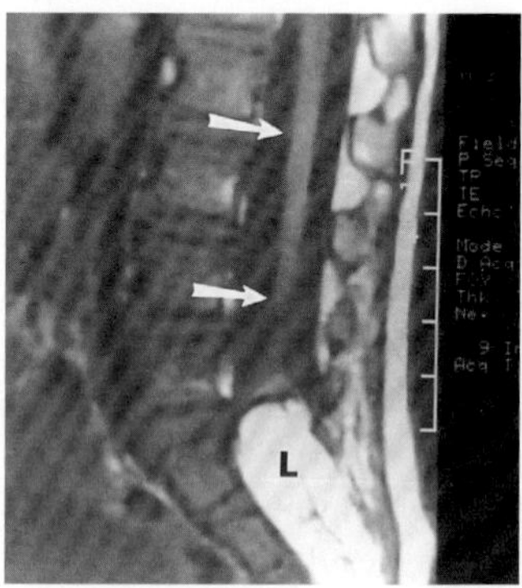

● **Figure 13-14 Tethered spinal cord.**

Case Study

After the delivery of a healthy baby girl, a physician noticed a tuft of hair on the child's lower back. The physician asked the mother about her prenatal health care, and she said she had not taken folic acid until the second month because she did not know she was pregnant until then.

Differentials

- Spina bifida occulta, spina bifida with meningocele, spina bifida with meningomyelocele

Relevant Physical Exam Findings

- Tuft of hair on physical observation
- No noticeable sac formation

Relevant Lab Findings

- X-ray confirms that there is a defect in the vertebral arches; however, it is negative for finding of a sac filled with fluid or spinal cord.

Diagnosis

- Spina bifida occulta is evidenced by the tuft of hair in the sacrolumbar region. Spina bifida of any type results from a lack of folic acid during the early period of pregnancy, that is, around day 28 of pregnancy.

Chapter **14**

Ear

I **Overview.** The ear is the organ of **balance** and **hearing**. The ear consists of an **internal ear**, a **middle ear**, and an **external ear**.

II **The Internal Ear (Figure 14-1; Table 14-1)** develops in **week 4** from a thickening of the surface ectoderm called the otic placode. The otic placode invaginates into the connective tissue (mesenchyme) adjacent to the rhombencephalon and becomes the otic vesicle. The otic vesicle divides into utricular and saccular portions.

A. UTRICULAR PORTION OF THE OTIC VESICLE gives rise to the:

1. **Utricle**
   a. Contains the sensory hair cells and otoliths of the macula utriculi.
   b. Responds to **linear acceleration** and the **force of gravity.**
2. **Semicircular ducts**
   a. Contain the sensory hair cells of the cristae ampullares.
   b. Respond to **angular acceleration.**
3. **Vestibular ganglion of CN VIII** lies at the base of the internal auditory meatus.
4. **Endolymphatic duct and sac**
   a. Is a membranous duct that connects the saccule to the utricle and terminates in a blind sac beneath the dura.
   b. The endolymphatic sac absorbs endolymph.

B. SACCULAR PORTION OF THE OTIC VESICLE gives rise to the:

1. **Saccule**
   a. Contains the sensory hair cells and otoliths of the macula sacculi.
   b. The saccule responds to **linear acceleration** and the **force of gravity**.
2. **Cochlear duct (organ of Corti)**
   a. Is involved in hearing.
   b. This duct has pitch (tonopic) localization by which high-frequency sound waves (20,000 Hz) are detected at the base and low-frequency sound waves (20 Hz) are detected at the apex.
   c. **Spiral ganglion of CN VIII** lies in the modiolus of the bony labyrinth.

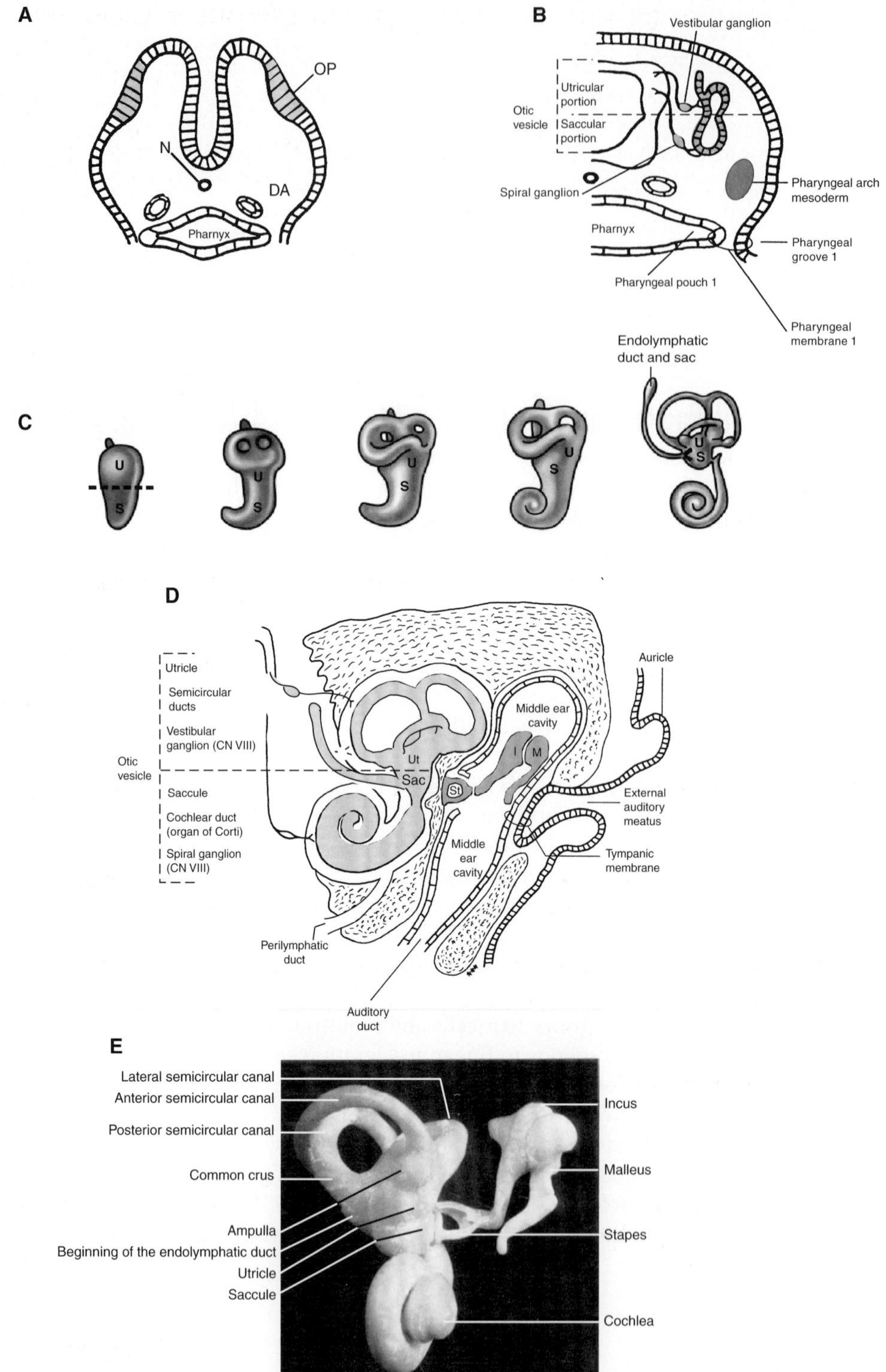

● **Figure 14-1 Schematic transverse sections showing the formation of the otic placode and otic vesicle from the surface ectoderm. (A)** The otic placode is distinguished by a thickening of the surface ectoderm. DA = dorsal aorta; N = notochord; OP = otic placode. **(B)** The otic placode invaginates into the underlying connective tissue (mesenchyme) and becomes the otic vesicle. **(C)** The otic vesicle undergoes extensive changes to form the adult membranous labyrinth. U = utricle; S = saccule. **(D)** The adult ear. M = malleus; I = incus; St = stapes. **(E)** The adult auditory ossicles in connection with the bony labyrinth (or internal ear).

TABLE 14-1 EMBRYONIC EAR STRUCTURES AND THEIR ADULT DERIVATIVES

Embryonic Structure	Adult Derivative
	Internal ear
Otic vesicle	
Utricular portion	Utricle, semicircular ducts, vestibular ganglion of CN VIII, endolymphatic duct and sac
Saccular portion	Saccule, cochlear duct (organ of Corti) spiral ganglion of CN VIII
	Middle ear
Pharyngeal arch 1	Malleus, incus, tensor tympani muscle
Pharyngeal arch 2	Stapes, stapedius muscle
Pharyngeal pouch 1	Auditory tube, middle ear cavity
Pharyngeal membrane 1	Tympanic membrane
	External ear
Pharyngeal groove 1	External auditory meatus
Auricular hillocks	Auricle

III The Membranous and Bony Labyrinths

A. The membranous labyrinth consists of all the structures derived from the otic vesicle (see Table14-1).

B. The membranous labyrinth is initially surrounded by neural crest cells that form a connective tissue (mesenchyme) covering. This connective tissue becomes cartilaginous and then ossifies to become the **bony labyrinth** of the temporal bone.

C. The connective tissue closest to the membranous labyrinth degenerates, thus forming the **perilymphatic space** containing **perilymph.**

D. This sets up the interesting anatomical relationship by which the membranous labyrinth is suspended (or floats) within the bony labyrinth by perilymph.

E. Perilymph, which is similar in composition to **cerebrospinal fluid** (CSF), communicates with the subarachnoid space via the **perilymphatic duct.**

IV The Middle Ear (Figure 14-1)

A. OSSICLES OF THE MIDDLE EAR

1. Malleus

a. Develops from cartilage of **pharyngeal arch 1** (Meckel's cartilage) and is attached to the tympanic membrane.

b. The malleus is moved by the **tensor tympani muscle**, which is innervated by CN V_3.

2. Incus

a. Develops from the cartilage of **pharyngeal arch 1** (Meckel's cartilage).

b. The incus articulates with the malleus and stapes.

3. Stapes

a. Develops from the cartilage of **pharyngeal arch 2** (Reichert's cartilage).

b. The stapes is moved by the **stapedius** muscle, which is innervated by CN VII.

c. Is attached to the oval window of the vestibule.

B. AUDITORY TUBE AND MIDDLE EAR CAVITY

1. Both of these structures develop from **pharyngeal pouch 1**.

C. TYMPANIC MEMBRANE

1. Develops from **pharyngeal membrane 1**.
2. This membrane separates the middle ear from the external auditory meatus of the external ear.
3. Is innervated by CN V_3 and CN IX.

V The External Ear (Figures 14-1 and 14-2)

A. EXTERNAL AUDITORY MEATUS

1. Develops from the **pharyngeal groove 1**.
2. The meatus becomes filled with ectodermal cells, forming a temporary **meatal plug** that disappears before birth.
3. The meatus is innervated by **CN V_3** and **CN IX**.

B. AURICLE (OR PINNA)

1. Develops from **six auricular hillocks** that surround pharyngeal groove 1.
2. The auricle is innervated by **CN V_3, CN VII, CN IX, and CN X** and **cervical nerves C_2 and C_3**.

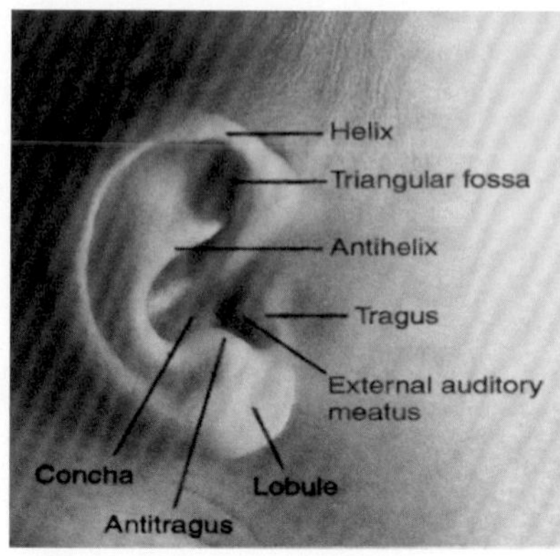

● Figure 14-2 The adult auricle.

VI Congenital Malformations of the Ear

A. MINOR AURICULAR MALFORMATIONS (FIGURE 14-3)

A. MINOR AURICULAR MALFORMATIONS (FIGURE 14-3) are commonly found and raise only cosmetic issues. However, auricular malformations are seen in **Down syndrome (trisomy 21), Patau syndrome (trisomy 13),** and **Edwards syndrome (trisomy 18).** Figure 14-3 shows a minor auricular variation called a cleft lobule (arrow).

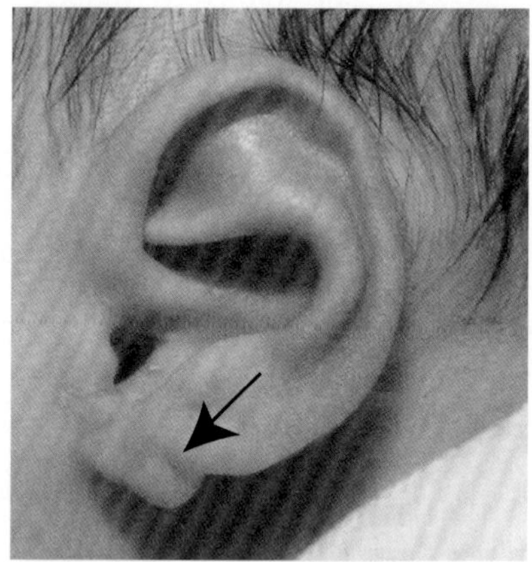

● Figure 14-3 Minor auricular malformation.

B. LOW-SET SLANTED AURICLES (FIGURE 14-4) are auricles that are located below a line extended from the corner of the eye to the occiput. This condition may indicate chromosomal abnormalities like **Down syndrome (trisomy 21)**, **Patau syndrome (trisomy 13)**, and **Edwards syndrome (trisomy 18)**. Figure 14-4 shows an infant with a severely low-set and posteriorly rotated auricle.

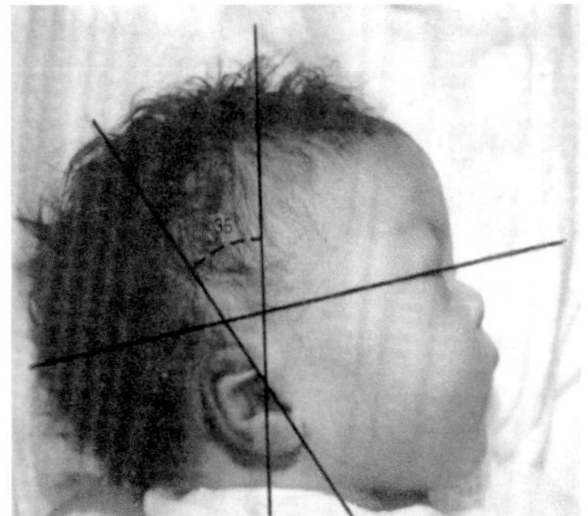

● **Figure 14-4 Low-set slanted auricles.**

C. AURICULAR APPENDAGES (FIGURE 14-5) are skin tags that are commonly found anterior to the auricle (i.e., pretragal area), which raise only cosmetic issues. The embryological basis is the formation of accessory auricle hillocks.

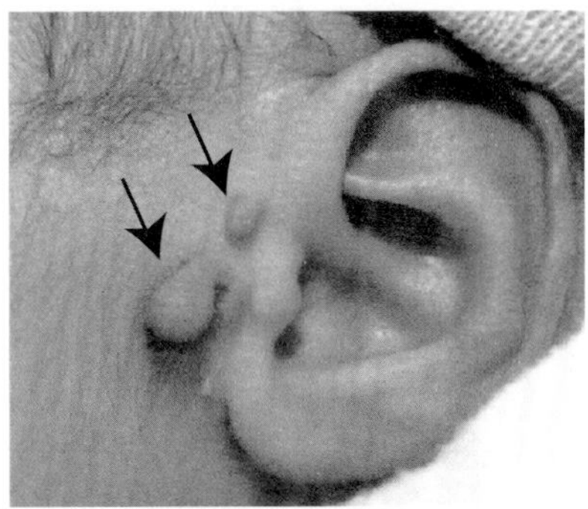

● **Figure 14-5 Auricular appendages.**

D. ATRESIA OF THE EXTERNAL AUDITORY MEATUS (FIGURE 14-6). A **complete atresia** consists of a bony plate in the location of the tympanic membrane. A **partial atresia** consists of a soft tissue plug in the location of the tympanic membrane. This results in conduction deafness and is usually associated with the first arch syndrome. The embryological basis is the failure of the meatal plug to canalize. Figure 14-6 shows the absence of the external auditory meatus in an infant.

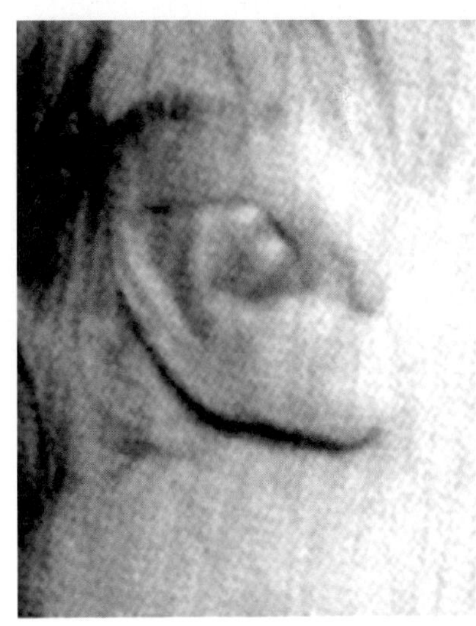

● **Figure 14-6 Atresia of the external auditory meatus.**

E. Preauricular sinus is a narrow tube or shallow pit that has a pinpoint external opening; it is most often asymptomatic and of minor cosmetic importance, although infections may occur. The embryological basis is uncertain, but probably involves pharyngeal groove 1.

F. CONGENITAL CHOLESTEATOMA (EPIDERMOID CYST) is a benign tumor found in the middle ear cavity that results in conduction deafness. The embryological basis is the proliferation of endodermal cells lining the middle ear cavity.

G. MICROTIA is a severely disorganized auricle that is associated with other malformations resulting in deafness. The embryological basis is impaired proliferation or fusion of the auricular hillocks.

H. CONGENITAL DEAFNESS. The organ of Corti may be damaged by exposure to **rubella virus**, especially during weeks 7 and 8 of development.

Case Study

A mother brings in her 1-week-old son to the clinic, stating that she "thinks her son can't hear her when she is calling to him." She remarks that while she was pregnant toward the beginning, she was ill and "broke out in a rash," but she thinks that "was due to a new lotion she was using." What is the most likely diagnosis?

Differentials

- Congenital hearing defect

Relevant Physical Exam Findings

- Microcephaly
- Deafness
- Hepatosplenomegaly

Relevant Lab Findings

- Low platelet count
- CSF was positive for rubella

Diagnosis

- Rubella

Chapter **15**

Eye

I Development of the Optic Vesicle (Figure 15-1; Table 15-1)

begins at day 22 with the formation of **optic sulcus**, which evaginates from the wall of the diencephalon as the **optic vesicle** consisting of **neuroectoderm**. The optic vesicle invaginates and forms a double-layered **optic cup** and **optic stalk**.

A. THE OPTIC CUP AND DERIVATIVES. The double-layered optic cup consists of an **outer pigment layer** and an **inner neural layer**.

1. Retina

a. The outer pigment layer of the optic cup gives rise to the **pigment layer of the retina.**

b. The **intraretinal space** separates the outer pigment layer from the inner neural layer. Although the intraretinal space is obliterated in the adult, it remains a weakened area prone to **retinal detachment**.

c. The inner neural layer of the optic cup gives rise to the **neural layer of the retina** (i.e., the rods and cones, bipolar cells, ganglion cells, etc).

2. Iris (Figure 15-2)

a. The epithelium of the iris develops from the anterior portions of both the outer pigment layer and the inner neural layer of the optic cup, which explains its histological appearance of two layers of columnar epithelium.

b. The stroma develops from mesoderm continuous with the choroid.

c. The iris contains the **dilator pupillae muscle** and **sphincter pupillae muscle**, which are formed from the epithelium of the outer pigment layer by a transformation of these epithelial cells into contractile cells.

3. Ciliary body (Figure 15-2)

a. The epithelium of the ciliary body develops from the anterior portions of both the outer pigment layer and the inner neural layer of the optic cup, which explains its histological appearance of two layers of columnar epithelium.

b. The stroma develops from mesoderm continuous with the choroid.

c. The ciliary body contains the **ciliary muscle**, which is formed from mesoderm within the choroid. The **ciliary processes** are components of the ciliary body.

d. The ciliary processes produce **aqueous humor**, which circulates through the posterior and anterior chambers and drains into the venous circulation via the **trabecular meshwork** and the **canal of Schlemm**.

e. The ciliary processes give rise to the **suspensory fibers** of the lens (ciliary zonule), which are attached to and suspend the lens.

B. THE OPTIC STALK AND DERIVATIVES

1. The optic stalk contains the **choroid fissure**, in which the **hyaloid artery and vein** are found. The hyaloid artery and vein later become the **central artery and vein of the retina**.
2. The optic stalk contains axons from the ganglion cell layer of the retina.

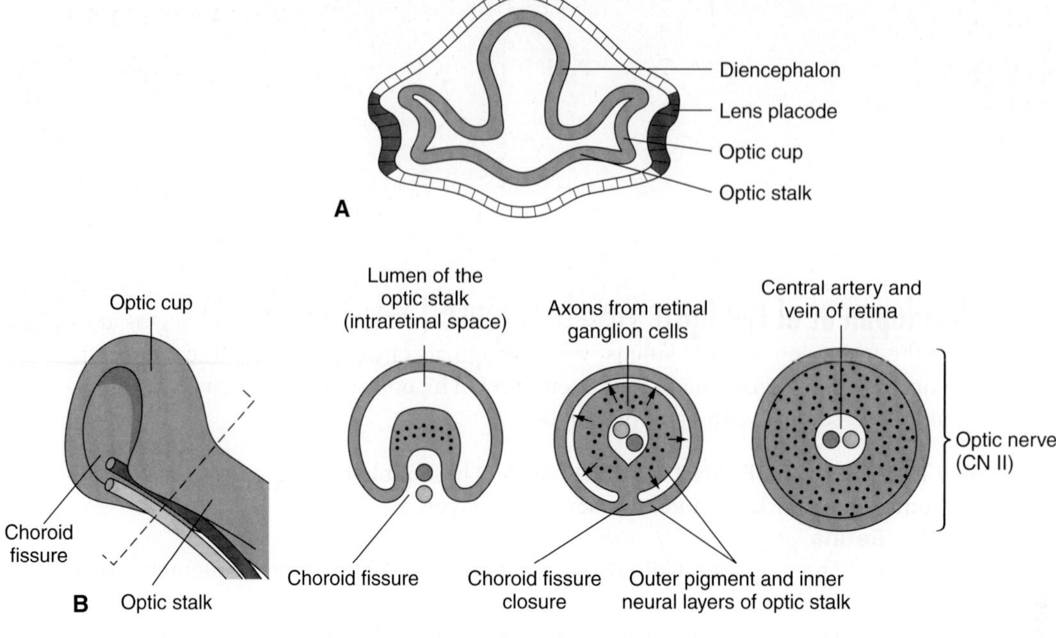

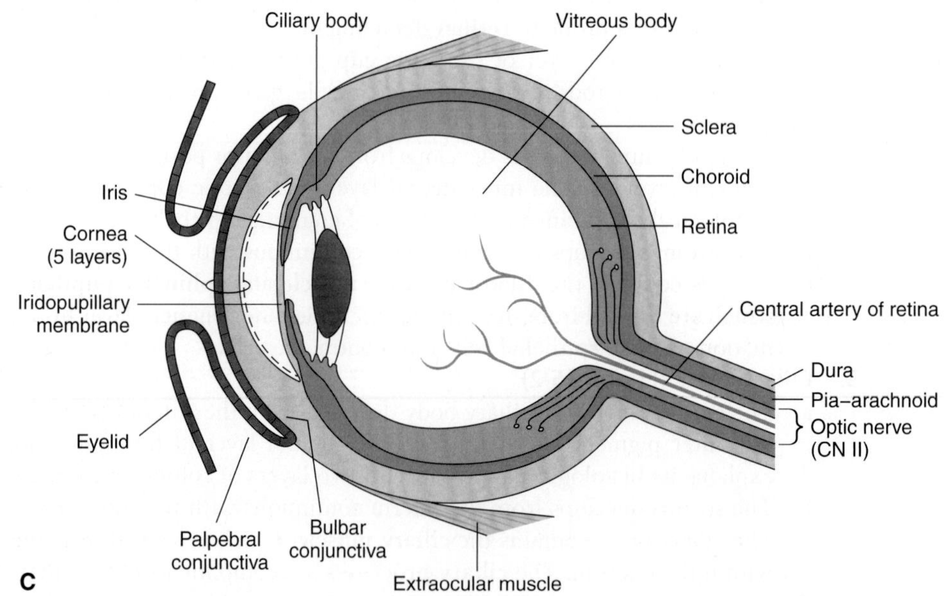

● **Figure 15-1 (A)** The optic cup and optic stalk are evaginations of the diencephalon. The optic cup induces surface ectoderm to differentiate into the lens placode. **(B)** Formation of the optic nerve (CN II) from the optic stalk. The choroid fissure, which is located on the undersurface of the optic stalk, permits access of the hyaloid artery and vein to the inner aspect of the eye. The choroid fissure eventually closes. As ganglion cells form in the retina, axons accumulate in the optic stalk and cause the inner and outer layers of the optic stalk to fuse, obliterating the lumen (or intraretinal space) and forming the optic nerve. **(C)** The adult eye. Note that the sclera is continuous with the dura mater and the choroid is continuous with the pia–arachnoid. The iridopupillary membrane is normally obliterated.

TABLE 15-1 EMBRYONIC EYE STRUCTURES AND THEIR ADULT DERIVATIVES

Embryonic Structure	Adult Derivative
Diencephalon (neuroectoderm)	
Optic cup	Retina, iris epithelium, dilator and sphincter pupillae muscles of iris, ciliary body epithelium
Optic stalk	Optic nerve (CN II), optic chiasm, optic tract
Surface ectoderm	Lens, anterior epithelium of cornea, bulbar and palpebral conjunctiva
Mesoderm	Sclera, choroid, stroma of iris, stroma of ciliary body, ciliary muscle, substantia propria of cornea, corneal endothelium, vitreous body, central artery and vein of retina, extraocular muscles

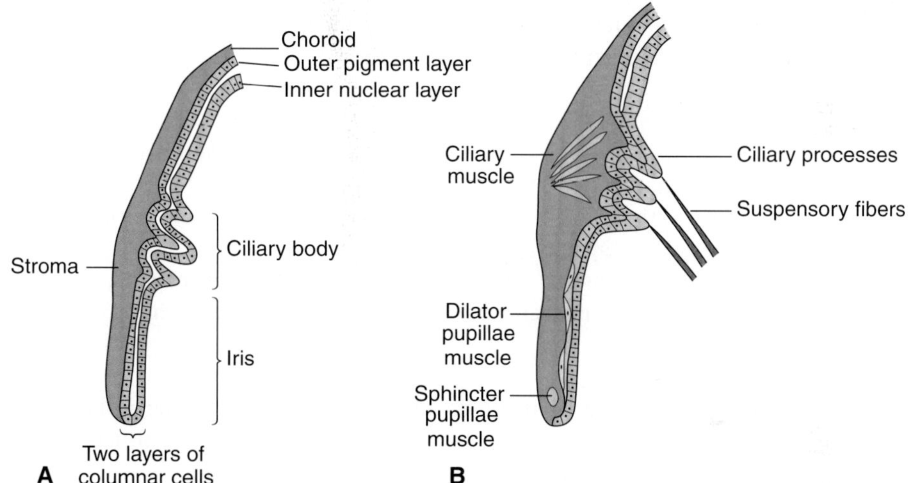

● **Figure 15-2 (A, B) Sagittal sections through the developing iris and ciliary body.** The iris and ciliary body form from the outer pigment layer and inner neural layer of the optic cup. In the adult, this embryological origin is reflected histologically by two layers of columnar epithelium that line both the iris and the ciliary body. Note the dilator and sphincter pupillae muscles associated with the iris and the ciliary muscle associated with the ciliary body.

3. The choroid fissure closes during week 7 so that the optic stalk, together with the axons of the ganglion cells, forms the **optic nerve (CN II), optic chiasm, and optic tract.**
4. The optic nerve (CN II) is a tract of the diencephalon and has the following characteristics:
   a. The optic nerve is not completely myelinated until 3 months after birth; it is myelinated by oligodendrocytes.
   b. The optic nerve is not capable of regeneration after transection.
   c. The optic nerve is invested by the meninges and therefore is surrounded by a subarachnoid space that plays a role in papilledema.

II Development of Other Eye Structures

A. SCLERA. The sclera develops from mesoderm surrounding the optic cup. The sclera forms an outer **fibrous** layer that is continuous with the dura mater posteriorly and the cornea anteriorly.

B. CHOROID. The choroid develops from mesoderm surrounding the optic cup. The choroid forms a **vascular** layer that is continuous with the pia/arachnoid posteriorly and iris/ciliary body anteriorly.

C. ANTERIOR CHAMBER. The anterior chamber develops from mesoderm over the anterior aspect of the eye that is continuous with the sclera and undergoes vacuolization to form a chamber. The anterior chamber essentially splits the mesoderm into two layers:

1. The mesoderm posterior to the anterior chamber is called the **iridopupillary membrane**, which is normally resorbed prior to birth.
2. The mesoderm anterior to the anterior chamber develops into the **substantia propria of the cornea** and **corneal endothelium**.

D. CORNEA

1. The cornea develops from both surface ectoderm and mesoderm lying anterior to the anterior chamber.
2. The surface ectoderm forms the **anterior epithelium of the cornea**, which has a high regenerative capacity.
3. The mesoderm forms the **substantia propria of the cornea** (i.e., **Bowman layer, stroma, and Descemet membrane**) and **corneal endothelium**.

E. LENS

1. The lens develops from surface ectoderm, which forms the **lens placode**.
2. The lens placode invaginates to form the **lens vesicle**. The adult lens is completely surrounded by a **lens capsule**.
3. The **lens epithelium** is a simple cuboidal epithelium located beneath the capsule only on the anterior surface.

F. VITREOUS BODY

1. The vitreous body develops from mesoderm that migrates through the choroid fissure and forms a transparent gelatinous substance between the lens and the retina.
2. The vitreous body contains a portion of the **hyaloid artery**, which later obliterates to form the **hyaloid canal** of the adult eye.

G. CANAL OF SCHLEMM. The canal of Schlemm is found at the sclerocorneal junction called the **limbus** and drains the **aqueous humor** into the venous circulation. An obstruction of the canal of Schlemm results in increased intraocular pressure (**glaucoma**).

H. EXTRAOCULAR MUSCLES. The extraocular muscles develop from mesoderm of **somitomeres 1, 2, and 3** (also **called preoptic myotomes**) that surround the optic cup.

III Congenital Malformations of the Eye

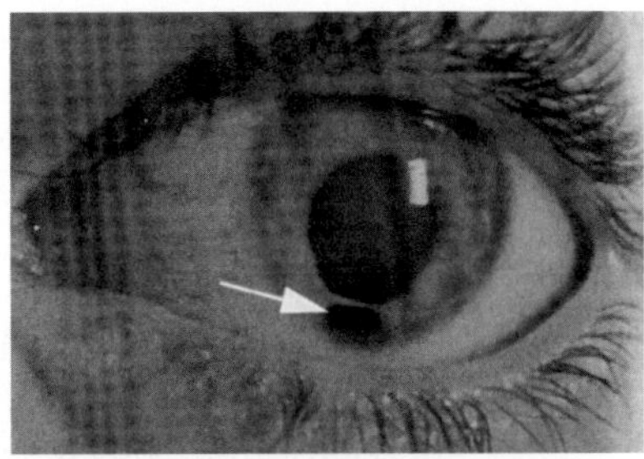

● **Figure 15-3 Coloboma iridis.**

A. COLOBOMA IRIDIS (FIGURE 15-3) is a cleft in the iris caused by failure of the choroid fissure to close in week 7 of development and may extend into the ciliary body, retina, choroid, or optic nerve. A **palpebral coloboma**—a notch in the eyelid—results from a defect in the developing eyelid. Figure 15-3 shows a cleft in the iris (black spot at arrow).

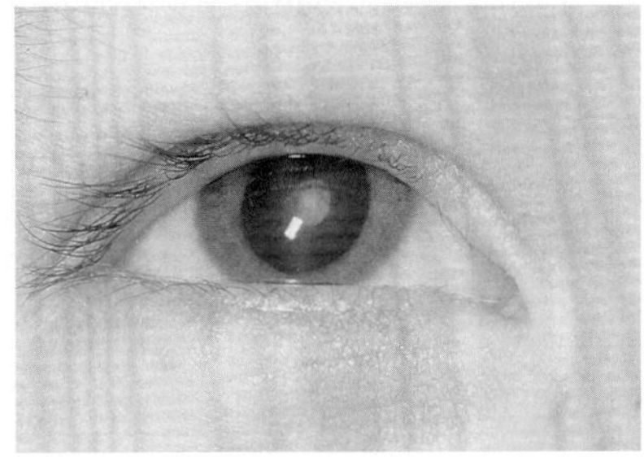

● **Figure 15-4 Congenital cataracts.**

B. CONGENITAL CATARACTS (FIGURE 15-4) are opacities of the lens and are usually bilateral. They are fairly common and may result from the following: rubella virus infection, toxoplasmosis, congenital syphilis, Down syndrome (trisomy 21), or galactosemia (an inborn error of metabolism). Figure 15-4 shows an infant with congenital cataracts. Note the lens opacity, indicating a polar cataract. Lens opacities in infants may be isolated or associated with a systemic condition. The morphology of infantile cataracts is distinctive, which differentiates infantile cataracts from other forms of cataracts. The location of the opacity in the eye of the infant permits a classification into polar, zonular (lamellar), nuclear, sutural, or total.

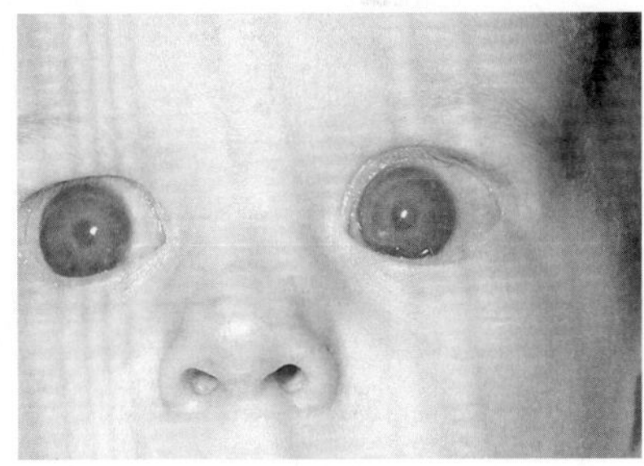

● **Figure 15-5 Congenital glaucoma (buphthalmos).**

C. CONGENITAL GLAUCOMA (BUPHTHALMOS) (FIGURE 15-5) is increased intraocular pressure due to abnormal development of the canal of Schlemm or the iridocorneal filtration angle. It is usually genetically determined, but may result from maternal rubella infection. Figure 15-5 shows enlarged right and left eyes. The dot reflex from the flash camera is not sharp. An enlarged eye is suspected when the corneal diameter exceeds 11 mm in a term newborn. If the eye is enlarged, infantile glaucoma caused by elevated intraocular pressure should be suspected immediately. Infantile glaucoma may also present with tearing, squinting, photosensitivity, and a cloudy cornea. The cornea often has horizontal lines called Haab striae, which result from a disruption of Descemet membrane.

D. PERSISTENT IRIDOPUPILLARY MEMBRANE (FIGURE 15-6) consists of strands of connective tissue that partially cover the pupil; however, it seldom affects vision. Figure 15-6 shows strands of connective tissue that partially cover the pupil.

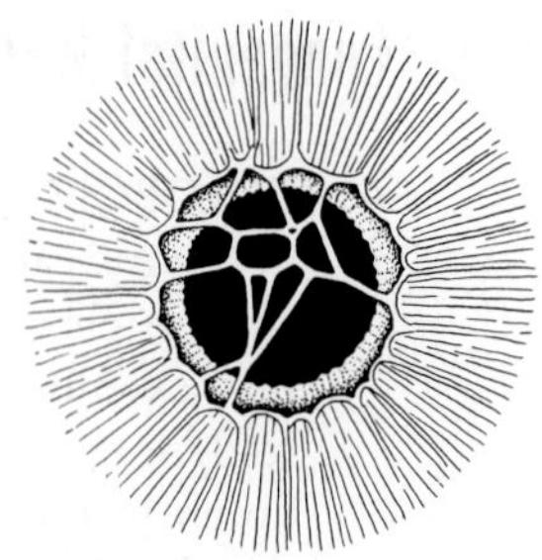

Figure 15-6 Persistent iridopupillary membrane.

E. RETINOBLASTOMA (RB) (FIGURE 15-7) is a tumor of the retina that occurs in childhood and develops from precursor cells in the immature retina. The RB gene is located on chromosome 13 and encodes for RB protein, which binds to a gene-regulatory protein and causes suppression of the cell cycle, that is, the RB gene is a **tumor-suppressor gene** (also called an **antioncogene**). A mutation in the RB gene will encode an abnormal RB protein such that there is no suppression of the cell cycle. This leads to the formation of RB. Hereditary RB causes multiple tumors in both eyes. Nonhereditary RB causes one tumor in one eye. In Figure 15-7, the computed tomography (CT) scan on the left shows multiple tumor calcifications (*arrows*) within the left intraorbital mass. The photograph on the right shows a large-sized RB that fills the entire eye.

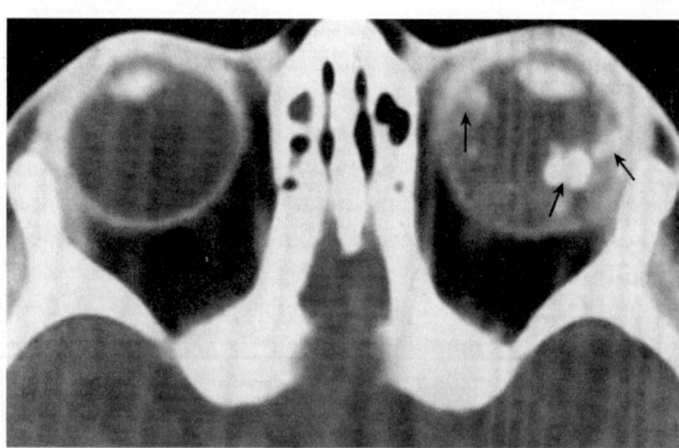

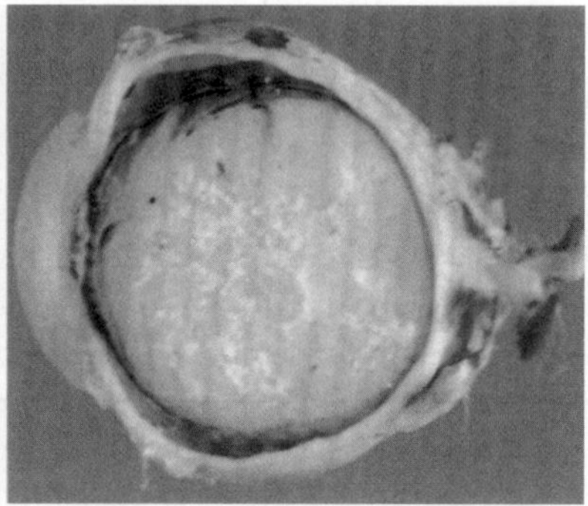

Figure 15-7 Retinoblastoma.

F. MICROPHTHALMIA is a small eye, usually associated with intrauterine infections from the TORCH group of microorganisms (*Toxoplasma*, rubella virus, cytomegalovirus, and herpes simplex virus).

G. ANOPHTHALMIA is absence of the eye. It is due to failure of the optic vesicle to form.

H. CYCLOPIA is a single orbit and one eye. It is due to failure of median cerebral structures to develop.

I. RETINOCELE results from herniation of the retina into the sclera or from failure of the choroid fissure to close.

J. **RETROLENTAL FIBROPLASIA** (retinopathy of prematurity) is an oxygen-induced retinopathy seen in premature infants.

K. **PAPILLEDEMA** is edema of the optic disk (papilla) due to increased intracranial pressure. This pressure is reflected into the subarachnoid space, which surrounds the optic nerve (CN II).

L. **RETINITIS PIGMENTOSA (RP)** is a hereditary degeneration and atrophy of the retina. RP may be transmitted as an autosomal recessive, autosomal dominant, or X-linked trait. RP is characterized by a degeneration of the rods, night blindness (nyctalopia), and "gun barrel vision." RP may also be due to abetalipoproteinemia (Bassen–Kornzweig syndrome), which may be arrested with massive doses of vitamin A.

Case Study

A young mother brings in her 3-year-old son because of "a white spot in his eye." She first noticed the spot in a photograph taken 2 weeks earlier. She remembers hearing about another family member with the same sort of spot, who eventually went blind. What is the most likely diagnosis?

Differentials
- Congenital cataract, congenital glaucoma, retinoblastoma

Relevant Physical Exam Findings
- Pupil with white spots
- Poor vision
- Crossed eyes

Relevant Lab Findings
- Genetic testing showing a mutation of the RB gene on chromosome 13

Diagnosis
- Retinoblastoma

Chapter **16**

Body Cavities

I Formation of the Intraembryonic Coelom (Figure 16-1)

A. The formation of the intraembryonic coelom begins when spaces coalesce within the lateral mesoderm and form a horseshoe-shaped space that opens into the chorionic cavity (extraembryonic coelom) on the right and left sides.

B. The intraembryonic coelom is remodeled due to the craniocaudal folding and lateral folding of the embryo.

C. The intraembryonic coelom can best be visualized as a balloon whose walls closest to the viscera are **visceral mesoderm** and whose walls closest to the body wall are **somatic mesoderm**.

D. The intraembryonic coelom provides the needed room for growth of various organs.

II Partitioning of the Intraembryonic Coelom (Figure 16-1).

The intraembryonic coelom is initially one continuous space. To form the definitive adult pericardial, pleural, and peritoneal cavities, two partitions must develop. The two partitions are the **paired pleuropericardial membranes** and the **diaphragm**.

A. PAIRED PLEUROPERICARDIAL MEMBRANES

1. Are sheets of somatic mesoderm that separate the **pericardial cavity** from the **pleural cavities.**
2. The formation of these membranes appears to be aided by lung buds invading the lateral body wall and by tension on the common cardinal veins resulting from rapid longitudinal growth.
3. These membranes develop into the definitive **fibrous pericardium** surrounding the heart.

B. DIAPHRAGM.

The diaphragm separates the **pleural cavities** from the **peritoneal cavity**. The diaphragm is formed through the fusion of tissue from four different sources:

1. **Septum transversum**
   a. Is a thick mass of mesoderm located between the primitive heart tube and the developing liver.
   b. The septum transversum is the primordium of the **central tendon of the diaphragm** in the adult.
2. **Paired pleuroperitoneal membranes** are sheets of somatic mesoderm that appear to develop from the dorsal and dorsolateral body wall by an unknown mechanism.
3. **Dorsal mesentery of the esophagus** is invaded by myoblasts and forms the **crura of the diaphragm** in the adult.
4. **Body wall** contributes muscle to the peripheral portions of the definitive diaphragm.

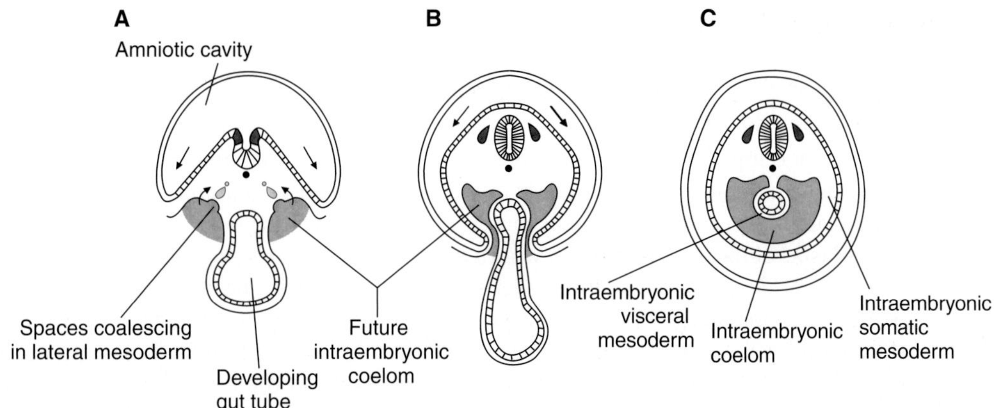

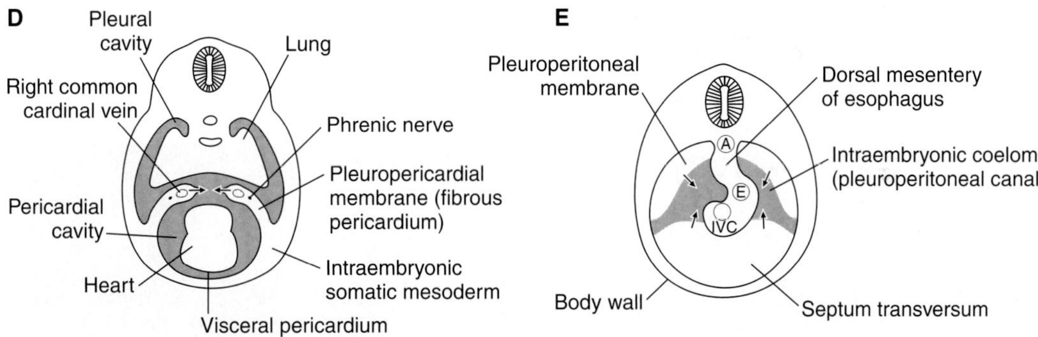

● **Figure 16-1 Diagram illustrating the formation and partitioning of the intraembryonic coelom (IC). (A, B, C)** Cross sections show various stages of IC formation while the embryo undergoes lateral folding. **(D)** Cross section shows two folds of intraembryonic somatic mesoderm carrying the phrenic nerves and common cardinal veins. The two folds fuse in the midline (*arrows*) to form the pleuropericardial membrane. This separates the pericardial cavity (*shaded*) from the pleural cavity (*shaded*). **(E)** Cross section of an embryo at week 5 shows the four components that fuse (*arrows*) to form the diaphragm, which closes off the IC between the pleural and peritoneal cavities. The portions of the IC that connect the pleural and peritoneal cavities in the embryo are called the pleuroperitoneal canals (*shaded*). A = aorta; E = esophagus; IVC = inferior vena cava.

III Positional Changes of the Diaphragm

A. During week 4 of development, the developing diaphragm becomes innervated by the **phrenic nerves**, which originate from C3, C4, and C5 and pass through the pleuropericardial membranes (this explains the definitive location of the phrenic nerves associated with the fibrous pericardium).

B. By week 8, there is an apparent **descent of the diaphragm to L1** because of the rapid growth of the neural tube. The phrenic nerves are carried along with the "descending diaphragm," which explains their unusually long length in the adult.

IV Clinical Considerations

A. **CONGENITAL DIAPHRAGMATIC HERNIA (FIGURE 16-2)** is a herniation of abdominal contents into the pleural cavity caused by a **failure of the pleuroperitoneal membrane** to develop or fuse with the other components of the diaphragm. A congenital diaphragmatic hernia is most commonly found on the **left posterolateral side** and is usually life threatening because abdominal contents compress the lung buds, causing **pulmonary hypoplasia**. Clinical signs in the newborn include: an unusually flat abdomen, breathlessness, severe dyspnea, peristaltic bowel sounds over the left chest, and cyanosis. It can be detected prenatally using ultrasonography. In Figure 16-2, the diagram on the left shows a congenital diaphragmatic hernia with herniation of intestinal loops into the left pleural cavity (*arrow*). The anteroposterior radiograph on the right shows a congenital diaphragmatic hernia. Note the loops of intestine within the pleural cavity as indicated by the bowel gas above and below the diaphragm and the mediastinal shift to the right.

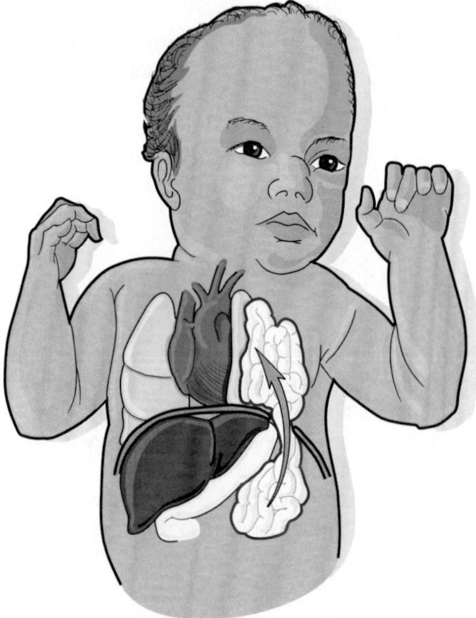

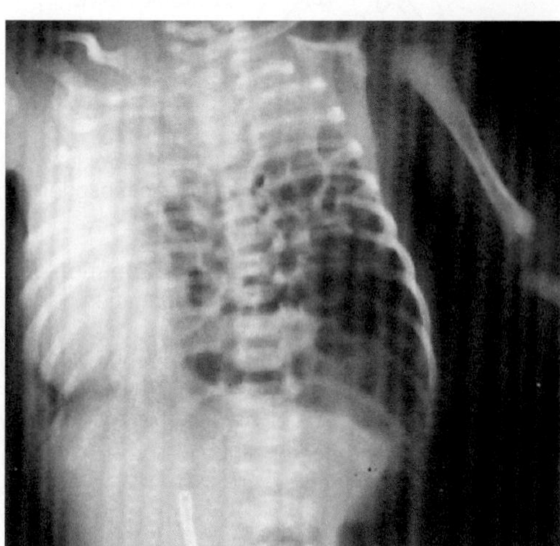

● **Figure 16-2 Congenital diaphragmatic hernia.**

B. **ESOPHAGEAL HIATAL HERNIA (FIGURE 16-3)** is a herniation of the stomach through the esophageal hiatus into the pleural cavity caused by an abnormally large esophageal hiatus. An esophageal hiatal hernia renders the **esophagogastric sphincter** incompetent so that stomach contents reflux into the esophagus. Clinical signs in the newborn include vomiting (frequently projectile) when the infant is laid on its back after feeding. Figure 16-3 shows an esophageal hiatal hernia. Note the large saccular, discolored, ischemic portion of the stomach (arrow) and the deviation of the esophagus to the right.

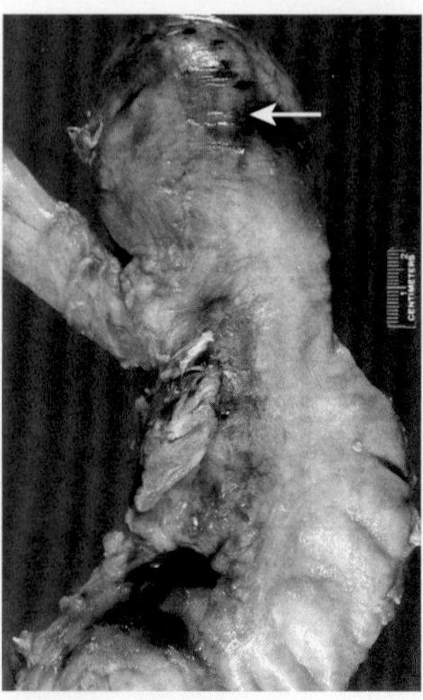

● **Figure 16-3 Esophageal hiatal hernia**

Case Study

The father of a 1-month-old daughter complains that she frequently "throws up after she eats," and "it just shoots across the room." What is the most likely diagnosis?

Differentials

- Pyloric stenosis, gastroesophageal reflux disease, esophageal hiatal hernia, congenital diaphragmatic hernia

Relevant Physical Exam Findings

- Projectile vomiting after the infant is laid on its back after a feeding

Relevant Lab Findings

- Chest radiograph shows herniation of the stomach through the esophageal hiatus into the pleural cavity.

Diagnosis

- Esophageal hiatal hernia

Chapter **17**

Pregnancy

I Endocrinology of Pregnancy (Figure 17-1)

A. HUMAN CHORIONIC GONADOTROPIN (hCG)

1. Overview

a. hCG is a glycoprotein hormone produced by the **syncytiotrophoblast**; it stimulates the production of progesterone (PG) by the corpus luteum (i.e., maintains corpus luteum function).

b. hCG can be assayed in **maternal blood at day 8** or **maternal urine at day 10** using a radioimmunoassay with antibodies directed against the β-subunit of hCG. This is the basis of the early pregnancy test kits purchased over the counter.

2. Quantitative hCG dating of pregnancy. During weeks 1–6 of a normal pregnancy, hCG levels will increase by about 70% every 48 hours:

a. 0–2 weeks: 0–250 mIU/mL
b. 2–4 weeks: 100–5000 mIU/mL
c. 1–2 months: 4000–200,000 mIU/mL
d. 2–3 months: 8000–100,000 mIU/mL
e. Second trimester: 4000–75,000 mIU/mL
f. Third trimester: 1000–5000 mIU/mL

3. Other tests using hCG

a. Low hCG levels may predict a spontaneous abortion or indicate an ectopic pregnancy.

b. Elevated hCG levels may indicate a multiple pregnancy, hydatidiform mole, or gestational trophoblastic neoplasia.

B. HUMAN PLACENTAL LACTOGEN (hPL)

1. hPL is a protein hormone produced by the **placenta**; it induces lipolysis, thereby elevating free fatty acid levels in the mother.

2. hPL is considered the "growth hormone" of the latter half of pregnancy.

3. hPL can be assayed in **maternal blood at week 6**.

4. hPL levels vary with placental mass (i.e., may indicate a multiple pregnancy) and rapidly disappear from maternal blood after delivery.

C. PROLACTIN (PRL)

1. PRL is a protein hormone produced by the **maternal adenohypophysis**, **fetal adenohypophysis**, and **decidual tissue of the uterus**; it prepares the mammary glands for lactation.

2. PRL can be assayed in **maternal blood throughout pregnancy** or later in **amniotic fluid**.

3. Near term, PRL levels rise to a maximum of about 100 ng/mL (normal nonpregnant PRL levels range between 8–25 ng/mL).

D. PROGESTERONE

1. **PG** is a steroid hormone produced by the **corpus luteum** until week 8 and then by the **placenta** until birth.
2. PG prepares the endometrium for implantation (nidation) and maintains the endometrium.
3. PG is used by the fetal adrenal cortex as a precursor for corticosteroid and mineralocorticoid synthesis.
4. PG is used by the fetal testes as a precursor for testosterone synthesis.

E. ESTRONE, ESTRADIOL, AND ESTRIOL

1. Little is known about the specific function of these steroid hormones in the mother or fetus during pregnancy. These steroid hormones are produced by complex series of steps involving the **maternal liver**, the **placenta**, and the **fetal adrenal gland** and **fetal liver** as follows:
   a. Cholesterol from the maternal liver is converted to pregnenolone by the placenta.
   b. Pregnenolone is converted to pregnenolone sulfate.
   c. Pregnenolone sulfate is converted to dehydroepiandrosterone sulfate (DHEA-SO_4) by the fetal adrenal gland.
   d. DHEA-SO_4 is converted to estrone and estradiol by the placenta.
   e. DHEA-SO_4 is also converted to 16α-hydroxy DHEA-SO_4 by the fetal liver.
   f. 16α-hydroxy DHEA-SO_4 is converted to estriol by the placenta.
2. **Estrone** is a fairly weak estrogen.
3. **Estradiol** is the most potent estrogen.
4. **Estriol**
   a. Estriol is a very weak estrogen but is produced in very high amounts during pregnancy.
   b. Estriol can be assayed in **maternal blood** (shows a distinct diurnal variation with peak amounts early in the morning) and **maternal urine** (24-hour urine sample shows no diurnal variation).
   c. Significant amounts of estriol are produced at month 3 (i.e., early second trimester) and continue to rise until birth.
   d. Maternal urinary levels of estriol have long been recognized as a **reliable index of fetal–placental function** because estriol production depends on a normal functioning fetal adrenal cortex, fetal liver, and placenta.

II Pregnancy Dating

A. The **estimated date of confinement (EDC)** is based on the assumption that a woman has a 28-day cycle with ovulation on day 14 or day 15.

B. In general, the duration of a normal pregnancy is **280 days (40 weeks) from the first day of the last menstrual period (LMP).**

C. A common method for determining the EDC (Naegele's rule) is to count back 3 months from the first day of the LMP and then add 1 year and 7 days. This method is reasonably accurate in women with regular menstrual cycles.

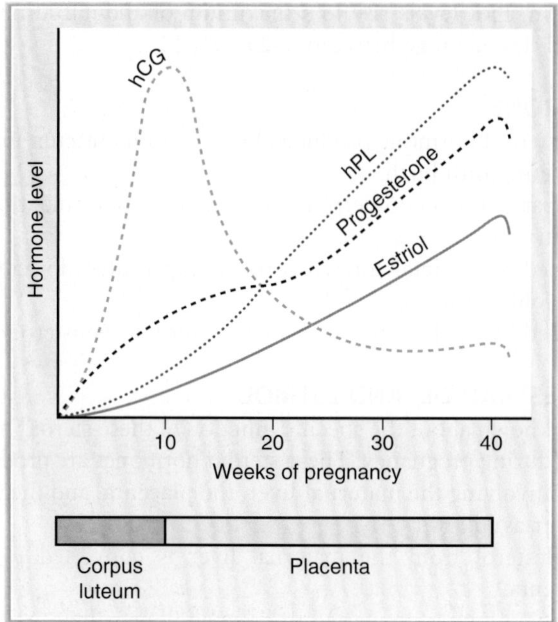

● **Figure 17-1 Hormone levels during pregnancy.** hCG = human chorionic gonadotropin; hPL = human placental lactogen.

III Pregnancy Milestones

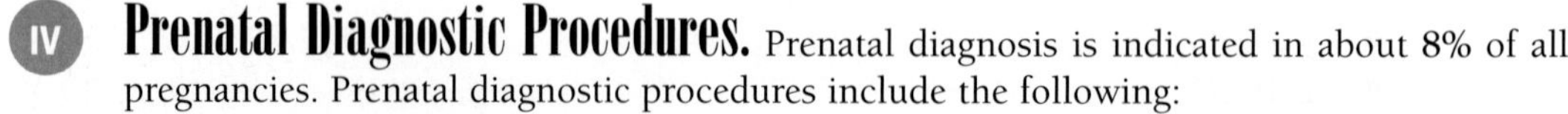

IV Prenatal Diagnostic Procedures.

Prenatal diagnosis is indicated in about 8% of all pregnancies. Prenatal diagnostic procedures include the following:

A. ULTRASONOGRAPHY

1. Ultrasonography is commonly used to date a pregnancy, to diagnose a multiple pregnancy, to assess fetal growth, to determine placenta location, to determine position and lie of the fetus, to detect certain congenital anomalies, and to monitor needle or catheter insertion during amniocentesis and chorionic villus biopsy.
2. In obstetric ultrasonography, 2.25- to 5.0-mHz frequencies are used for good tissue differentiation.
3. The term **anechoic** refers to tissues with few or no echoes (e.g., bladder, brain, cavities, amniotic fluid).
4. The term **echogenic** refers to tissues with a high capacity to reflect ultrasound.
5. **B scan ultrasonography** consists of an **A mode** and an **M mode** (which provide precise measurements) and a **time position scan** with a permanent record of cinephotography.
6. **Real-time ultrasonography** provides an easy, immediate, and definitive demonstration of fetal life.

B. AMNIOCENTESIS

1. Amniocentesis is a transabdominal sampling of **amniotic fluid** and **fetal cells**.
2. Amniocentesis is performed at weeks 14–18 and is indicated in the following situations: the woman is older than 35 years of age, a previous child has a chromosomal anomaly, one parent is a known carrier of a translocation or inversion, one or both parents are known carriers of an X-linked recessive or autosomal recessive trait, or there is a history of neural tube defects.

TABLE 17-1 PREGNANCY MILESTONES

Trimester	Events
First (from the last menstrual period through week 12)	At days 8–10, a positive pregnancy test is obtained by hCG assay. At week 12, the uterine fundus is palpable at the pubic symphysis Doppler fetal heart rate is first audible.
Second (from end of the first trimester through week 27)	At weeks 14–18, amniocentesis is performed when suspicion of fetal chromosomal abnormalities exists. At week 16, uterine fundus is palpable midway between the pubic symphysis and umbilicus. At weeks 16–18, first fetal movements occur (quickening) in a woman's second or higher pregnancy. At weeks 17–20, fetal heart rate is audible with the fetoscope. At week 18, female and male external genitalia can be distinguished by ultrasound (i.e., sex determination). At weeks 18–20, first fetal movements occur (quickening) in a woman's first pregnancy. At week 20, uterine fundus is palpable at the umbilicus. At weeks 25–27, lungs become capable of respiration; surfactant is produced by Type II pneumocytes. There is a 70%–80% chance of survival in infants born at the end of the second trimester. If death occurs, it is generally as a result of lung immaturity and resulting hyaline membrane disease. At week 27, the fetus weighs about 1000 g (a little more than 2 lb).
Third (from end of second trimester until term or week 40)	Pupillary light reflex is present. Descent of the fetal head to the pelvic inlet (called lightening) occurs. Rupture of the amniochorionic membrane occurs, with labor usually beginning about 24 hours later. The fetus weighs about 3300 g (about 7–7.5 lb).

3. The sample obtained is used in the following studies:
   a. **α-Fetoprotein assay** is used to diagnose neural tube defects.
   b. **Spectrophotometric assay of bilirubin** is used to diagnose hemolytic disease of the newborn (i.e., erythroblastosis fetalis) due to Rh-incompatibility.
   c. **Lecithin–sphingomyelin (L/S) ratio and phosphatidylglycerol assay** are used to determine lung maturity of the fetus.
   d. **DNA analysis:** A wide variety of DNA methodologies is available (e.g., karyotype analysis, Southern blotting, or RFLP [restriction fragment length polymorphism] analysis) to diagnose chromosomal abnormalities and single-gene defects.

C. CHORIONIC VILLUS BIOPSY

1. Chorionic villus biopsy is a transabdominal or transcervical sampling of the chorionic villi to obtain a large amount of **fetal cells** for DNA analysis.

2. Chorionic villus biopsy is performed at weeks 6–11 (i.e., much earlier than amniocentesis), thereby providing an early source of fetal cells for DNA analysis.

D. PERCUTANEOUS UMBILICAL BLOOD SAMPLING (PUBS) is a sampling of fetal blood from the umbilical cord.

V Fetal Distress During Labor (Intrapartum)

A. Fetal distress during labor is defined in terms of **fetal hypoxia** and measured by changes in either **fetal heart rate (FHR)** or **fetal scalp capillary pH.**

B. The normal baseline FHR is 120–160 beats per minute. However, fetal hypoxia causes a decrease in FHR (or **fetal bradycardia**), that is, a **FHR <120 beats per minute**.

C. The normal fetal scalp capillary pH is 7.25–7.35. However, fetal hypoxia causes a decrease in pH, that is, a **pH <7.20**.

VI The APGAR Score (Table 17-2)

A. The APGAR score assesses five characteristics (appearance, pulse, grimace, activity, respiratory effort) in the newborn infant to determine which infants need resuscitation.

B. The APGAR score is calculated at 1 minute and again at 5 minutes after birth.

C. To obtain an APGAR score, one scores 0, 1, or 2 for the five characteristics and adds them together.

1. **APGAR score of 0–3** indicates a life-threatening situation.
2. **APGAR score of 4–6** indicates temperature and ventilation support is needed.
3. **APGAR score of 7–10** indicates a normal situation.

TABLE 17-2 ASSESSING THE APGAR SCORE

	Score			
Characteristic	**0**	**1**	**2**	**Clinical Example**
Appearance, color	Blue, pale	Body pink, extremities blue	Completely pink	1
Pulse, heart rate	Absent	<100 beats per minute	>100 beats per minute	2
Grimace, reflex, irritability	No response	Grimace	Vigorous crying	0
Activity, muscle tone	Flaccid	Some flexion of extremities	Active motion, flexed extremities	0
Respiratory effort	None	Weak, irregular	Good, crying	1
APGAR score				**4**

Clinical example: A newborn infant at 5 minutes after birth has a pink body but blue extremities (score 1); a heart rate of 125 beats per minute (score 2); shows no grimace or reflex (score 0); has flaccid muscle tone (score 0); and has weak irregular breathing (score 1). The total APGAR score is 4. This infant needs ventilation and temperature support.

VII Puerperium

A. Puerperium extends from immediately after delivery of the baby until the reproductive tract returns to the nonpregnant state in approximately 4–6 weeks.

B. Important events that occur are:

1. Involution of the uterus
2. Afterpains due to uterine contractions
3. Uterine discharge (lochia)
4. In nonlactating women, menstrual flow returns within 6–8 weeks postpartum, and ovulation returns 2–4 weeks postpartum.
5. In lactating women, ovulation may return within 10 weeks postpartum. Birth control protection afforded by lactation is assured for only 6 weeks, after which time pregnancy is possible.

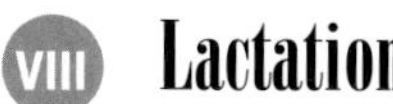

VIII Lactation

A. LACTATION DURING PREGNANCY

1. hPL, PRL, PG, estrogens, cortisol, and insulin stimulate the growth of **lactiferous ducts** and proliferation of epithelial cells to form **alveoli.**
2. Alveoli secrete **colostrum.**

B. LACTATION AFTER DELIVERY OF THE BABY

1. Lactation is initiated by a decrease in PG and estrogens, along with the release of PRL from the adenohypophysis.
2. This initiates **milk production.**

C. LACTATION DURING SUCKLING

1. A stimulus from the breast inhibits the release of PRL-inhibiting factor from the hypothalamus, thereby causing a **surge in PRL**, which increases milk production.
2. In addition, stimulation of the nipples during suckling causes a **surge of oxytocin,** which causes the expulsion of accumulated milk ("milk letdown") by stimulating myoepithelial cells.

Chapter 18
Teratology

I Introduction (Figure 18-1).

A teratogen is any infectious agent, drug, chemical, or irradiation that alters fetal morphology or fetal function if the fetus is exposed during a critical stage of development.

A. RESISTANT PERIOD (WEEK 1 OF DEVELOPMENT). The resistant period (week 1 of development) is the time when the conceptus demonstrates the "all-or-none" phenomenon—that is, the conceptus will either die as a result of the teratogen or survive unaffected.

B. MAXIMUM SUSCEPTIBILITY PERIOD (WEEKS 3–8). The maximum susceptibility period (weeks 3–8; embryonic period) is the time when the embryo is most susceptible to teratogens because all organ morphogenesis occurs at this time.

C. LOWERED SUSCEPTIBILITY PERIOD (WEEKS 9–38; FETAL PERIOD). The lowered susceptibility period (weeks 9–38; fetal period) is the time when the fetus has a lowered susceptibility to teratogens because all organ systems have already formed; generally results in a *functional* derangement of an organ system.

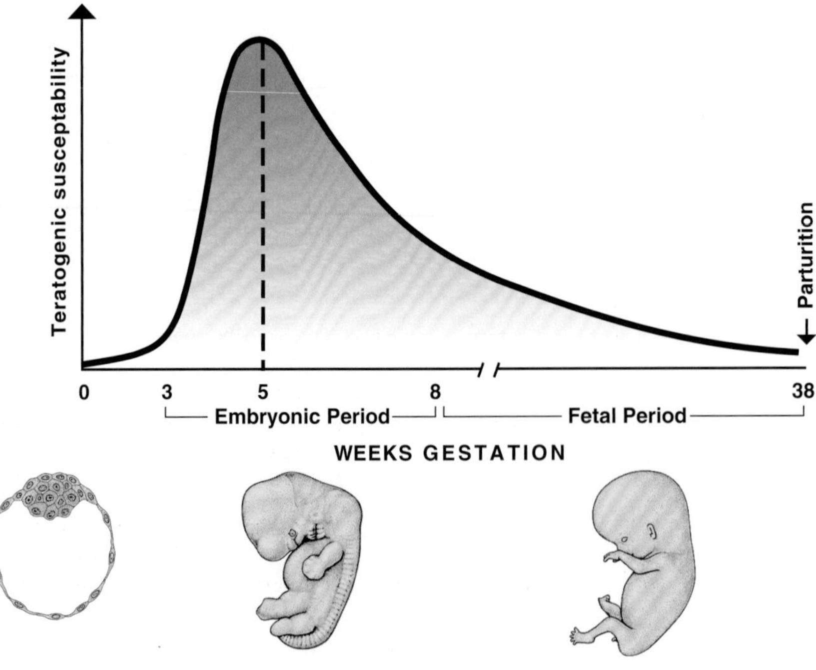

● **Figure 18-1** Critical stages of teratogenic susceptibility.

II Infectious Agents

Infectious Agents may be viral or nonviral. However, bacteria appear to be nonteratogenic.

A. VIRAL INFECTIONS may reach the fetus via the amniotic fluid following vaginal infection, transplacentally via the bloodstream after maternal viremia, or by direct contact during passage through an infected birth canal.

1. **Rubella virus (German measles; member of TORCH)**
   a. The rubella virus belongs to the **Togaviridae** family, which are **enveloped, icosahedral, positive single-stranded RNA viruses.**
   b. The rubella virus is transmitted to the fetus **transplacentally.**
   c. The risk of fetal rubella infection is greatest during the **first month of pregnancy** and apparently declines thereafter.
   d. Fetal rubella infection results in the classic triad of **cardiac defects** (patent ductus arteriosus, pulmonary artery stenosis, atrioventricular [AV] septal defects), **cataracts**, and **low birth weight.**
   e. The clinical manifestations include intrauterine growth retardation (most common manifestation), hepatosplenomegaly, generalized adenopathy, hemolytic anemia, hepatitis, jaundice, meningoencephalitis, eye involvement (e.g., cataracts, glaucoma, retinopathy), bluish-purple lesions on a yellow, jaundiced skin ("blueberry muffin spots"), osteitis (celery-stalk appearance of long bones), and sensorineural deafness.
   f. Control measures for rubella prevention should be placed on immunization of children.
2. **Cytomegalovirus (CMV; member of TORCH)**
   a. CMV belongs to the **Herpesvirus** family, which are **large, enveloped, icosahedral, double-stranded DNA viruses.** CMV is a ubiquitous virus and the **most common fetal infection.**
   b. CMV is transmitted to the fetus **transplacentally**, with more severe malformations when infection occurs during the first half of pregnancy. CMV is also transmitted to perinates **during passage through the birth canal or through breast milk** but causes no apparent disease.
   c. The most common manifestation of CMV fetal infection is **sensorineural deafness.**
   d. **Cytomegalic inclusion disease** (characterized by multiorgan involvement) is the most serious but least common manifestation of CMV infection and results in intrauterine growth retardation, microcephaly, chorioretinitis, hepatosplenomegaly, osteitis (celery-stalk appearance of long bones), discrete cerebral calcifications, mental retardation, heart block, and bluish-purple lesions on a yellow, jaundiced skin ("blueberry muffin spots").
3. **Herpes simplex virus (HSV-1; HSV-2; member of TORCH)**
   a. HSV belongs to the **Herpesvirus** family, which are **large, enveloped, icosahedral, double-stranded DNA viruses.** Most neonatal infections are caused by HSV-2 (75% of the cases).
   b. HSV-2 is transmitted to the fetus **transplacentally** only occasionally (5% of the cases). HSV-2 is most commonly transmitted to the fetus by **direct contact during passage through an infected birth canal** (intrapartum; 85% of cases).
   c. **At 10–11 days of age**, some intrapartum HSV-infected infants present with the disease localized to the **skin** (discrete vesicular lesion, large bullae, or denuded skin; hallmark signs), **eye** (keratoconjunctivitis, uveitis, chorioretinitis,

cataracts, retinal dysplasia), or **mouth** (ulcerative lesions of the mouth, tongue, or palate).

d. **At 15–17 days of age**, some intrapartum HSV-infected infants present with **central nervous system (CNS) involvement** (with or without skin, eye, or mouth involvement) due to axonal retrograde transport of HSV to the brain. Clinical manifestations of CNS involvement include lethargy, bulging fontanelles, focal or generalized seizures, opisthotonus, decerebrate posturing, and coma.
e. **At 9–11 days of age**, some intrapartum HSV-infected infants present with **disseminated disease**. Clinical manifestations of disseminated disease include CNS, liver, adrenal gland, pancreas, and kidney involvement due to hematogenous spread of HSV.
f. The only intervention shown to prevent neonatal HSV infection is delivery by cesarean section within 4–6 hours of rupture of the amnionic membranes.

4. **Varicella zoster virus (VZV; varicella or chickenpox)**
   a. **VZV** belongs to the **Herpesvirus** family, which are **large, enveloped, icosahedral, double-stranded DNA viruses.**
   b. VZV is transmitted to the fetus **transplacentally** in 25% of the cases, but **fetal varicella syndrome** develops only when maternal VZV infection occurs in the first trimester.
   c. The clinical manifestations of fetal varicella syndrome include cicatricial (scarring) skin lesions in a dermatomal pattern, limb and digit hypoplasia, limb paresis/paralysis, hydrocephalus, microcephaly/mental retardation, seizures, chorioretinitis, and cataracts.
   d. Administration of the live, attenuated VZV vaccine to susceptible women *before* pregnancy and to their susceptible household members (older than 1 year) is the most effective method of prevention.
5. **Human immunodeficiency virus (HIV)**
   a. HIV belongs to the **Retroviridae** family (or **Lentivirus** subfamily), which are **diploid, enveloped, positive single-stranded RNA viruses.**
   b. HIV is believed by many investigators to be the major cause of **acquired immunodeficiency syndrome (AIDS)**. However, others believe that multiple blood transfusions (e.g., in hemophiliacs), consumption of megadoses of antibiotics as prophylaxis against sexually transmitted diseases, and continuous use of drugs to heighten orgasm (e.g., amyl and butyl nitrite) destroy $CD4^+$ T cells and lead to AIDS.
   c. The placenta is a highly effective barrier to HIV infection of the fetus. However, HIV is transmitted to the fetus **through blood containing HIV or HIV-infected lymphoid cells** near the time of delivery or after 35 weeks of gestation.
   d. HIV infection does not appear to cause any congenital malformations, but results in chronic, multisystem infections.
   e. The clinical manifestations include **fungal infections** (e.g., *Candida* esophagitis, *Cryptococcal* meningitis, histoplasmosis, coccidioidomycosis, *Pneumocystis carinii* pneumonia), **bacterial infections** (e.g., *Mycobacterium* tuberculosis, *Mycobacterium avium-intracellulare* complex infection, *Streptococcus pneumoniae* infection, gastroenteritis caused by *Salmonella*, *Shigella*, and *Campylobacter*), **viral infections** (e.g., HSV-1, HSV-2, and CMV), and protozoan infections (e.g., *Cryptosporidium*, *Giardia*, *Toxoplasma,* and *Entamoeba*).

B. NONVIRAL INFECTIONS

1. *Toxoplasma gondii* (TG; member of TORCH)

a. TG is a **protozoan parasite** whose life cycle is divided into a **sexual phase** that occurs only in cats (**the definitive host**) and an **asexual phase** that occurs in intermediate hosts.

b. Generally speaking, mice that eat cat feces contaminate fields, thereby infecting cows, sheep, and pigs. TG is transmitted to humans primarily through ingestion of oocyst-containing water or food or consumption of oocyst-containing raw or undercooked meat. In addition, inhalation or ingestion of oocysts from soil, dust, or a cat litter box may occur.

c. TG is transmitted to the fetus **transplacentally** in 25%, 54%, and 65% of pregnant women with untreated primary toxoplasmosis during the first, second, and third trimesters, respectively.

d. TG infection results in miscarriage, perinatal death, chorioretinitis, microcephaly, hydrocephalus, and encephalomyelitis with cerebral calcification.

2. *Treponema pallidum* (TP)

a. TP is a **spirochete** causing **syphilis.**

b. TP is transmitted to the fetus **transplacentally** in 10%, 40%, 50%, and 50% of pregnant women with a late latent stage, early latent stage, primary stage, and secondary stage of syphilis, respectively. The most important determinant of risk to the fetus is the maternal stage of syphilis.

c. Infection acquired at birth through contact with a genital lesion in the birth canal may also occur but is rare.

d. TP infection results in miscarriage, perinatal death, hepatosplenomegaly, hepatitis, joint swelling, vesiculobullous blisters whose fluid contains active spirochetes and is highly infective, nasal discharge with rhinitis, a maculopapular rash located on the extremities that is initially oval and pink, but then turns copper brown and desquamate (palm and soles), eye findings (including chorioretinitis, glaucoma, cataracts, and uveitis), anemia, jaundice, focal erosions of the proximal medial tibia (Wimberger sign), osteitis (celery-stalk appearance of long bones), saw-toothed appearance of the metaphysis of long bones, abnormal teeth (Hutchinson teeth), acute syphilitic leptomeningitis, which may present as neck stiffness, and chronic meningovascular syphilis (cranial nerve palsy, hydrocephalus, cerebral infarction).

III TORCH Infections

TORCH Infections are caused by *Toxoplasma* (T), **rubella** (R), **cytomegalovirus** (C), **herpesvirus** (H), and **other** (O) bacterial and viral infections that are grouped together because they cause similar clinical and pathological manifestations.

IV Category X Drugs (Absolute Contraindication in Pregnancy)

A. THALIDOMIDE is an **antinauseant** drug that was prescribed for pregnant women (no longer used) for "morning sickness." This drug can cause limb reduction (e.g., meromelia, amelia), ear and nasal abnormalities, cardiac defects, lung defects, pyloric or duodenal stenosis, and gastrointestinal atresia.

B. AMINOPTERIN AND METHOTREXATE are **folic acid antagonists** used in cancer chemotherapy. These drugs can cause small stature, abnormal cranial ossification, ocular hypertelorism, low-set ears, cleft palate, and myelomeningocele.

C. **BUSULFAN (MYLERAN), CHLORAMBUCIL (LEUKERAN), CYCLOPHOSPHAMIDE (CYTOXAN)** are **alkylating agents** used in cancer chemotherapy. These drugs can cause cleft palate, eye defects, hydronephrosis, renal agenesis, absence of toes, and growth retardation.

D. **PHENYTOIN (DILANTIN)** is an **antiepileptic** drug. In 30% of cases, this drug causes **fetal hydantoin syndrome**, which results in growth retardation, mental retardation, microcephaly, craniofacial defects, and nail and digit hypoplasia. In the majority of cases, this drug causes cleft lip, cleft palate, and congenital heart defects.

E. **TRIAZOLAM (HALCION) AND ESTAZOLAM (PROSOM)** are hypnotic drugs. These drugs can cause cleft lip and cleft palate, especially if used in the first trimester of pregnancy.

F. **WARFARIN (COUMADIN)** is an **anticoagulant** drug that acts by inhibiting vitamin K–dependent coagulation factors. This drug can cause stippled epiphyses, mental retardation, microcephaly, seizures, fetal hemorrhage, and optic atrophy in the fetus. Note the mnemonic <u>war</u>farin causes WAR on the fetus.

G. **ISOTRETINOIN (ACCUTANE)** is a **retinoic acid derivative** used in the treatment of **severe acne.** This drug can cause CNS abnormalities, external ear abnormalities, eye abnormalities, facial dysmorphia, and cleft palate (i.e., **vitamin A embryopathy**).

H. **CLOMIPHENE (CLOMID)** is a **nonsteroidal ovulatory stimulant** used in women with ovulatory dysfunction. Although no causative evidence of a deleterious effect of clomiphene on the human fetus has been established, there have been reports of birth anomalies.

I. **DIETHYLSTILBESTROL (DES)** is a **synthetic estrogen** that was used to prevent spontaneous abortion in women. This drug can cause cervical hood, T-shaped uterus, hypoplastic uterus, ovulatory disorders, infertility, premature labor, and cervical incompetence in women who were exposed to DES in utero. These women are also subject to increased risk of adenocarcinoma of the vagina later in life.

J. **ETHISTERONE, NORETHISTERONE, AND MEGESTROL (MEGACE)** are synthetic **progesterone derivatives.** These drugs can cause masculinization of genitalia in female embryos, hypospadias in males, and cardiovascular anomalies.

K. **OVCON, LEVLEN, AND NORINYL** are **oral contraceptives** that contain a combination of estrogen (e.g., ethinyl estradiol or mestranol) and progesterone (e.g., norethindrone or levonorgestrel) derivatives. These drugs can cause an increase of fetal abnormalities, particularly the **VACTERL syndrome** consisting of vertebral, anal, cardiac, tracheoesophageal, renal, and limb malformations.

L. **NICOTINE** is a **poisonous, addictive alkaloid** delivered to the fetus through **cigarette smoking** by pregnant women (cigarette smoke also contains **hydrogen cyanide** and **carbon monoxide**). This drug can cause intrauterine growth retardation, premature delivery, low birth weight, and fetal hypoxia due to reduced uterine **blood flow and diminished capacity** of the blood to transport oxygen to fetal tissue.

M. **ALCOHOL** is an **organic compound** delivered to the fetus through **recreational or addictive (i.e., alcoholism) drinking** by pregnant women. This drug can cause **fetal alcohol syndrome**, which results in mental retardation, microcephaly, holoprosencephaly, limb deformities, craniofacial abnormalities (i.e., hypertelorism, long philtrum, and short palpebral fissures), and cardiovascular defects (i.e., ventricular septal defects). Fetal alcohol syndrome is the leading cause of mental retardation.

V Category D Drugs (Definite Evidence of Risk to Fetus)

A. **TETRACYCLINE (ACHROMYCIN) AND DOXYCYCLINE (VIBRAMYCIN)** are **antibiotics** in the tetracycline family. These drugs can cause permanently stained teeth and hypoplasia of enamel.

B. **STREPTOMYCIN, AMIKACIN, AND TOBRAMYCIN (NEBCIN)** are **antibiotics** in the aminoglycoside family. These drugs can cause **CN VIII toxicity** with permanent bilateral deafness and loss of vestibular function.

C. **PHENOBARBITAL (DONNATAL) AND PENTOBARBITAL (NEMBUTAL)** are **barbiturates** used as **sedatives.** Studies have suggested a higher incidence of fetal abnormalities with maternal barbiturate use.

D. **VALPROIC ACID (DEPAKENE)** is an **antiepileptic** drug. This drug can cause neural tube defects, cleft lip, and renal defects.

E. **DIAZEPAM (VALIUM), CHLORDIAZEPOXIDE (LIBRIUM), ALPRAZOLAM (XANAX), AND LORAZEPAM (ATIVAN)** are **anticonvulsant** or **antianxiety** drugs. These drugs can cause cleft lip and cleft palate, especially if used in the first trimester of pregnancy.

F. **LITHIUM** is used in treatment of **manic-depressive disorder.** This drug can cause fetal cardiac defects (i.e., Ebstein's anomaly and malformations of the great vessels).

G. **CHLOROTHIAZIDE (DIURIL)** is a **diuretic** and **antihypertensive** drug. This drug can cause fetal jaundice and thrombocytopenia.

VI Chemical Agents

A. **ORGANIC MERCURY.** Consumption of organic mercury during pregnancy results in fetal neurological damage, including seizures, psychomotor retardation, cerebral palsy, blindness, and deafness.

B. **LEAD.** Consumption of lead during pregnancy results in abortion due to embryotoxicity, growth retardation, increased perinatal mortality, and developmental delay.

C. **POLYCHLORINATED BIPHENYLS (PCBS).** Consumption of PCBs during pregnancy results in intrauterine growth retardation, dark-brown skin pigmentation, exophthalmos, gingival hyperplasia, skull calcification, mental retardation, and neurobehavioral abnormalities.

D. **BISPHENOL A** is a common ingredient in plastics used to make reusable water bottles and in resins used to line food cans and dental sealants. Bisphenol A has been associated with higher rates of breast cancer in animal studies.

E. **PHTHALATES** are a common ingredient in vinyl flooring, detergents, automotive plastics, soap, shampoo, deodorants, hair sprays, blood storage bags, and intravenous medical tubing. High phthalate levels in pregnant women have been associated with testicular changes in their infant sons, leading to lower concentrations of male hormones and incomplete testicular descent. Phthalates have antiandrogenic activity.

F. PERFLUOROOCTANOIC ACID (PFOA) is a common ingredient of stain-, grease-, and water-resistant plastics like Teflon and Gore-Tex. PFOA is a likely carcinogen associated with liver, breast, pancreatic, and testicular cancers.

G. METHOXYCHLOR (AN INSECTICIDE) AND VINCLOZOLIN (A FUNGICIDE) are considered "endocrine disruptors." Recent studies have shown that the exposure of pregnant mice to either of these chemicals affected not just the male offspring exposed in utero, but all males for the next four subsequent generations.

H. POTASSIUM IODIDE (PI) is found in over-the-counter cough medicines and radiograph cocktails for organ visualization and is involved in thyroid enlargement (goiter) and mental retardation (cretinism).

VII Recreational Drugs

A. LYSERGIC ACID (LSD) has not been shown to be teratogenic.

B. MARIJUANA has not been shown to be teratogenic.

C. CAFFEINE has not been shown to be teratogenic.

D. COCAINE results in an increased risk of various congenital abnormalities, stillbirths, low birth weight, and placental abruption.

E. HEROIN has not been shown to be teratogenic. It is drugs that are often taken with heroin that produce congenital anomalies. The principal adverse effect is **severe neonatal withdrawal**, causing death in 3%–5% of neonates. **Methadone** (used to replace heroin) is not teratogenic, but is also associated with severe neonatal withdrawal.

VIII Ionizing Radiation

A. ACUTE HIGH DOSE (>250 RADS) results in microcephaly, mental retardation, growth retardation, and leukemia. After exposure to **greater than 25 rads**, classic fetal defects will be observed, so that termination of pregnancy should be offered as an option. Much information concerning acute high-dose radiation has come from studies of the atomic explosions over Hiroshima and Nagasaki.

B. DIAGNOSTIC RADIATION. Even if several radiographic studies are performed, rarely does the dose add up to significant exposure to produce fetal defects. **Radioactive iodine cocktails** for organ visualization should be avoided after week 10 of gestation because fetal thyroid development can be impaired.

IX Selected Photographs

A. TORCH INFECTIONS (FIGURE 18-2)

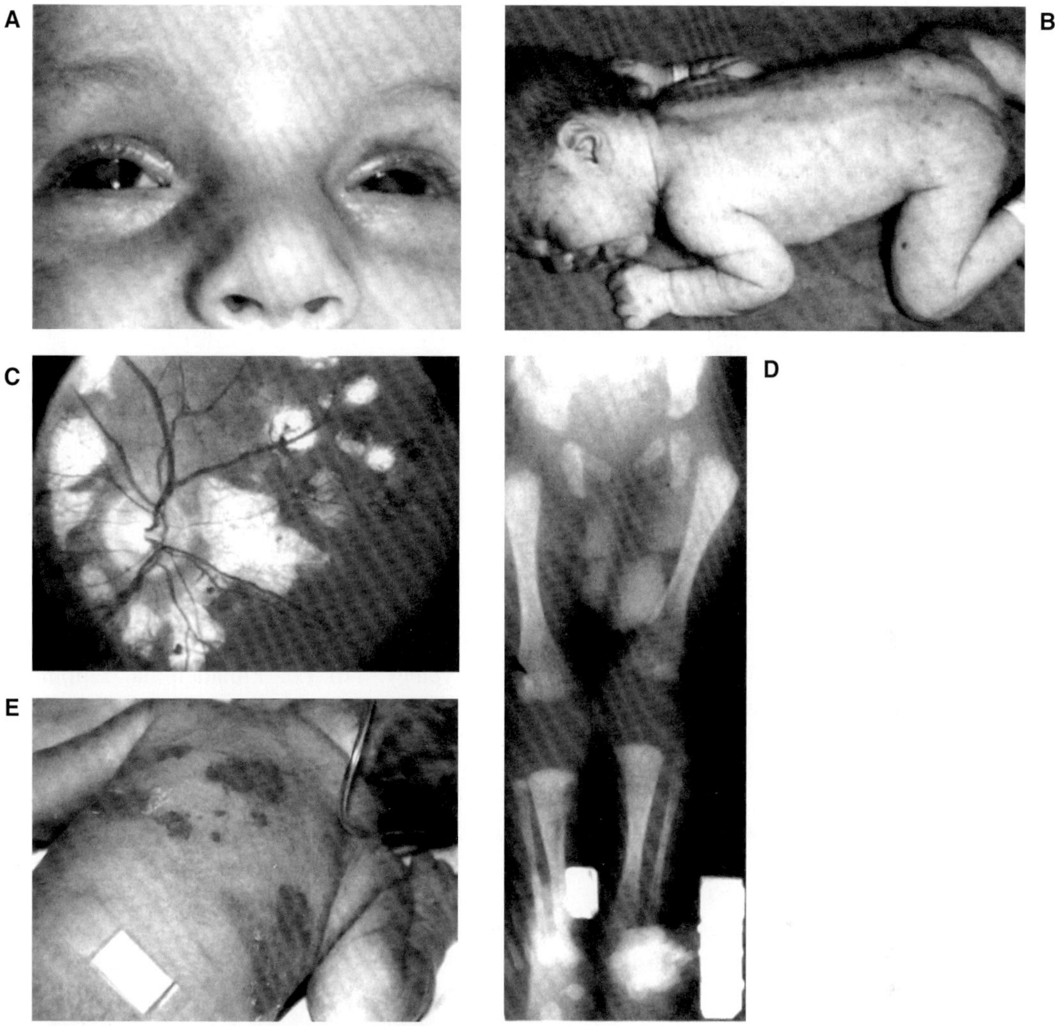

A

B

C

D

E

F

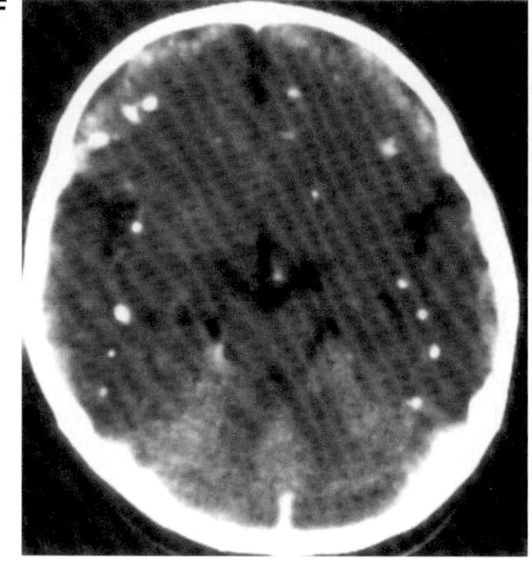

● **Figure 18-2 TORCH infections. (A)** Cataracts seen with congenital rubella and herpes simplex virus infections. **(B)** Blueberry muffin spots seen with congenital rubella and cytomegalovirus infections due to extramedullary hematopoiesis. **(C)** Patchy, yellow-white lesions of chorioretinitis seen with congenital cytomegalovirus, herpes simplex virus, and *Toxoplasma gondii* infections. **(D)** Celery-stalk appearance of the femur (*arrowhead*) and tibia seen with congenital rubella, cytomegalovirus, and syphilis infections. The alternating bands of longitudinal translucency and density indicate a disturbance in normal bone metabolism. **(E)** Cutaneous vesicular lesions surrounded by an erythematous border on the back and right arm seen with congenital herpes simplex virus infection. **(F)** Diffuse cerebral calcifications seen with congenital cytomegalovirus and *Toxoplasma gondii* infections.

Credits

Figure 1-1: Adapted from Dudek RW, Fix JD. *Board Review Series: Embryology*. 2nd Ed. Philadelphia: Lippincott Williams & Wilkins, 1998:4.

Figure 1-2: From Dudek RW. *High-Yield Histology*. 3rd Ed. Philadelphia: Lippincott Williams & Wilkins, 2004:218.

Figure 1-3: Adapted from Dudek RW, Fix JD. *Board Review Series: Embryology*. 2nd Ed. Philadelphia: Lippincott Williams & Wilkins, 1998:4.

Figure 3-2: Adapted from Sternberg SS. *Diagnostic Surgical Pathology*. Vol. 2. 3rd Ed. Philadelphia: Lippincott Williams & Wilkins, 1999.

Figure 3-3: Adapted from Sternberg SS. *Diagnostic Surgical Pathology*. Vol. 2. 3rd Ed. Philadelphia: Lippincott Williams & Wilkins, 1999.

Figure 4-2: Courtesy of Dr. Don Nakayama, Department of Surgery, University of North Carolina.

Figure 4-3: From Sadler TW. *Langman's Medical Embryology*. 7th Ed. Philadelphia: Lippincott Williams & Wilkins, 1995:61,62.

Figure 5-2: From Dudek RW, Fix JD. *Board Review Series: Embryology*. 3rd Ed. Philadelphia: Lippincott Williams & Wilkins, 2005:26.

Figure 5-3: From Dudek RW, Fix JD. *Board Review Series: Embryology*. 3rd Ed. Philadelphia: Lippincott Williams & Wilkins, 2005:54.

Figure 6-2: From Dudek RW. *Board Review Series: Embryology*. 3rd Ed. Philadelphia: Lippincott Williams & Wilkins, 2005:34.

Figure 6-3: From Dudek RW. *Board Review Series: Embryology*. 3rd Ed. Philadelphia: Lippincott Williams & Wilkins, 2005:36. **Radiograph:** From McMillan JA, DeAngelis CD, Feigin RD, et al., eds. *Oski's Pediatrics: Principles and Practice*. 3rd Ed. Philadelphia: Lippincott Williams & Wilkins, 1999:1349.

Figure 6-4: From Dudek RW. *Board Review Series: Embryology*. 3rd Ed. Philadelphia: Lippincott Williams & Wilkins, 2005:37. **Radiograph b1:** From Kirks DR, Griscom NT. *Practical Pediatric Imaging*. 3rd Ed. Philadelphia: Lippincott Williams & Wilkins, 1998:555. **Radiograph d1.** From Kirks DR, Griscom NT. *Practical Pediatric Imaging*. 3rd Ed. Philadelphia: Lippincott Williams & Wilkins, 1998:553.

Figure 6-5: From Dudek RW. *Board Review Series: Embryology*. 3rd Ed. Philadelphia: Lippincott Williams & Wilkins, 2005:38. **Radiograph:** From Kirks DR, Griscom NT. *Practical Pediatric Imaging*. 3rd Ed. Philadelphia: Lippincott Williams & Wilkins, 1998:519. **Venticulograph:** From McMillan JA, DeAngelis CD, Feigin RD, et al., eds. *Oski's Pediatrics: Principles and Practice*. 3rd Ed. Philadelphia: Lippincott Williams & Wilkins, 1999:1356.

Figure 7-2: (**A**) From Fenoglio-Preiser CM, Noffsinger AE, Stemmermann GE, et al., eds. *Gastrointestinal Pathology: An Atlas and Text*. 2nd Ed. Philadelphia: Lippincott Williams & Wilkins, 1998:33. (**B**) Fenoglio-Preiser CM, Fenoglio-Preiser CM, Noffsinger AE, Stemmermann GE, et al., eds. *Gastrointestinal Pathology: An Atlas and Text*. 2nd Ed. Philadelphia: Lippincott Williams & Wilkins, 1998:37. Courtesy of Dr. Cooley Butler, Scripps Memorial Hospital, La Jolla, CA.

Figure 7-3: **(A)** From Johnson KE. *NMS Human Developmental Anatomy*. Baltimore: Williams & Wilkins, 1988:211. **(B)** From Yamada T, Alpers DH, Laine L, et al., eds. *Textbook of Gastroenterology*. Vol. 1. 3rd Ed. Philadelphia: Lippincott Williams & Wilkins, 1999:1337.

Figure 7-4: From Johnson KE. *NMS Human Developmental Anatomy*. Baltimore: Williams & Wilkins, 1988:215.

Figure 7-5: **(A,B)** Modified from Cubilla AL, Fitzgerald PJ. Tumors of the exocrine pancreas. In: Hartmann WH, Sobin LH, eds. *Atlas of Tumor Pathology*, 2nd series, fascicle 19. Washington, DC: Armed Forces Institute of Pathology, 1984. **(C)** From Dudek RW. *High-Yield Systems Gastrointestinal Tract*. Philadelphia: Lippincott Williams & Wilkins, 2010:10. **Original source:** From Swischuk LE. *Imaging of the Newborn, Infant, and Young Child.* 5th Ed. Philadelphia: Lippincott Williams & Wilkins, 2004:392.

Figure 7-6: **(A)** From Johnson KE. *NMS Human Developmental Anatomy*. Baltimore: Williams & Wilkins, 1988:218. **(B–D)** From Fenoglio-Preiser CM, Noffsinger AE, Stemmermann GE, et al., eds. *Gastrointestinal Pathology: An Atlas and Text*. 2nd Ed. Philadelphia: Lippincott Williams & Wilkins, 1998:311, 312. **(E)** From Swischuk LE. *Imaging of the Newborn, Infant, and Young Child.* 5th Ed. Philadelphia: Lippincott Williams & Wilkins, 2004:410.

Figure 7-7: **(A)** From Sternberg SS. *Histology for Pathologists*. 2nd Ed. Baltimore: Williams & Wilkins, 1997:554. **(B)** From Swischuk LE. *Imaging of the Newborn, Infant, and Young Child.* 5th Ed. Philadelphia: Lippincott Williams & Wilkins, 2004:448.

Figure 8-1: From *Dudek RW. Board Review Series: Embryology*. 4th Ed. Philadelphia: Lippincott Williams & Wilkins, 2008:148.

Figure 8-2: From Dudek RW. *Board Review Series: Embryology*. 4th Ed. Philadelphia: Lippincott Williams & Wilkins, 2008:148.

Figure 8-3: From Kirks DR, Griscom NT. *Practical Pediatric Imaging*. 3rd Ed. Philadelphia: Lippincott Williams & Wilkins, 1998.

Figure 8-4: From Kirks DR, Griscom NT. *Practical Pediatric Imaging*. 3rd Ed. Baltimore: Williams & Wilkins, 1998.

Figure 8-5: From Avery GB. *Neonatology: Pathophysiology and Management of the Newborn*. 5th Ed. Philadelphia: Lippincott Williams & Wilkins, 1999:979.

Figure 8-6: From Dudek RW. *Board Review Series: Embryology*. 4th Ed. Philadelphia: Lippincott Williams & Wilkins, 2008:152.

Figure 8-7: From Sternberg SS. *Histology for Pathologists*, vol. 2. 3rd Ed. Baltimore: Williams & Wilkins, 1999:1827.

Figure 8-8: From Eisenberg RL. *Clinical Imaging*. 4th Ed. Philadelphia: Lippincott Williams & Wilkins, 2003:301.

Figure 9-1: **(A–C)** Adapted from Shakzkes DR, Haller JO, Velcek FT. Imaging of uterovaginal anomalies in the pediatric population. *Urol Radiol* 1991;13:58. With kind permission of Springer Science + Business Media. **(D,E)** From Dudek RW, Fix JD. *Board Review Series: Embryology*. 3rd Ed. Philadelphia: Lippincott Williams & Wilkins, 2005:151.

Figure 9-2: **(A,B)** From Dudek RW, Fix JD. *Board Review Series: Embryology*. 3rd Ed. Philadelphia: Lippincott Williams & Wilkins, 2005:152. **(C)** From Fletcher MA. *Physical Diagnosis in Neonatology*. Philadelphia: Lippincott-Raven, 1998:369. **(D)** From Sternberg SS. *Histology for Pathologists*. 2nd Ed. Philadelphia: Lippincott Williams & Wilkins, 1999:852.

Figure 9-3: From Janovski NA. Ovarian tumors. In: Friedman EA, ed. *Major Problems in Obstetrics and Gynecology*. Vol. 4. Philadelphia: WB Saunders, 1973:191.

Figure 9-5: **Radiograph** from Fleischer AC. *Clinical Gynecologic Imaging*. Philadelphia: Lippincott Williams & Wilkins, 1998:304.

Figure 9-6: **Radiographs** from Berek JS. *Novak's Gynecology*. 13th Ed. Philadelphia: Lippincott Williams & Wilkins, 2002:818. Courtesy of Dr. A Gerbie. From Spitzer IB, Rebar RW. Counseling for women with medical problems: ovary and reproductive organs. In: Hollingsworth D, Resnik R, eds. *Medical Counseling before Pregnancy*. New York: Churchill Livingstone, 1988: 213–248.

Figure 9-7: Radiograph from Berek JS. *Novak's Gynecology*. 13th Ed. Philadelphia: Lippincott Williams & Wilkins, 2002:818. Courtesy of Dr. A Gerbie. From Spitzer IB, Rebar RW. Counseling for women with medical problems: ovary and reproductive organs. In: Hollingsworth D, Resnik R, eds. *Medical Counseling before Pregnancy*. New York: Churchill Livingstone, 1988:213–248.

Figure 9-9: Left radiograph. From Gidwani G. *Congenital Malformation of the Female Genital Tract*. Philadelphia: Lippincott Williams & Wilkins, 1999:81.

Right radiograph. From Moore KL, Dalley AF. *Clinically Oriented Anatomy*. 5th Ed. Philadelphia: Lippincott Williams & Wilkins, 2006:469.

Figure 10-1: (**A–C**) From Shakzkes DR, Haller JO, Velcek FT. Imaging of uterovaginal anomalies in the pediatric population. *Urol Radiol* 1991;13:58. With kind permission of Springer Science + Business Media. Markham SM, Waterhouse TB. Structural anomalies of the reproductive tract. *Curr Opin Obstet Gynecol* 1992;4:867. (**D,E**) From Dudek RW, Fix JD. *Board Review Series: Embryology*. 3rd Ed. Philadelphia: Lippincott Williams & Wilkins, 2005:160.

Figure 10-2: From Dudek RW, Fix JD. *Board Review Series: Embryology*. 3rd Ed. Philadelphia: Lippincott Williams & Wilkins, 2005:161.

Figure 10-3: (**A**) From Sadler TW. *Langman's Medical Embryology*. 9th Ed. Philadelphia: Lippincott Williams & Wilkins, 2004:352. Courtesy of Dr. R. J. Gorlin, Department of Oral Pathology and Genetics, University of Minnesota. (**B**) Courtesy of Dr. T. Ernesto Figueroa, Wilmington, Delaware.

Figure 10-4: From MacDonald MG, Mullett MD, Seshia MM, eds. *Avery's Neonatology: Pathophysiology and Management of the Newborn*. 5th Ed. Philadelphia: Lippincott Williams & Wilkins, 2005:995.

Figure 10-5: From Fletcher MA. *Physical Diagnosis in Neonatology*. Philadelphia: Lippincott-Raven, 1998:378.

Figure 10-6: Courtesy of Dr. T. Ernesto Figueroa, Wilmington, Delaware.

Figure 10-7: From Sadler TW. *Langman's Medical Embryology*. 9th Ed. Philadelphia: Lippincott Williams & Wilkins, 2004.

Figure 10-8: From Warkany J. *Congenital Malformations: Notes and Comments*. Chicago: Year Book Medical Publishers, 1971:337.

Figure 10-9: From Jones HW, Scott WW. *Hermaphroditism, Genital Anomalies and Related Endocrine Disorders*. Baltimore: Williams & Wilkins, 1958:119.

Figure 11-1: Adapted from Dudek RW, Fix JD. *Board Review Series: Embryology*. 3rd Ed. Philadelphia: Lippincott Williams & Wilkins, 2005:119.

Figure 11-2: From Yamada T, Alpers DH, Laine L, et al., eds. *Textbook of Gastroenterology*. Vol. 1. 3rd Ed. Philadelphia: Lippincott Williams & Wilkins, 1999:1186.

Figure 11-3: From Rohen JW, Yokochi C, Lutjen-Drecoll E, et al. *Color Atlas of Anatomy*. 4th Ed. Philadelphia: Lippincott Williams & Wilkins, 1998:235.

Figure 11-4: From Kirks DR, Griscom NT. *Practical Pediatric Imaging*. 3rd Ed. Philadelphia: Lippincott Williams & Wilkins, 1998.

Figure 11-5: From Kirks DR, Griscom NT. *Practical Pediatric Imaging*. 3rd Ed. Philadelphia: Lippincott Williams & Wilkins, 1998.

Figure 11-6: (**A**) From Dudek RW, Fix JD. *Board Review Series: Embryology*. 3rd Ed. Philadelphia: Lippincott Williams & Wilkins, 2005:124. (**B**) From Kirks DR, Griscom NT. *Practical Pediatric Imaging*. 3rd Ed. Philadelphia: Lippincott Williams & Wilkins, 1998:695.

Figure 12-1: From Dudek RW, Fix JD. *Board Review Series: Embryology*. 3rd Ed. Philadelphia: Lippincott Williams & Wilkins, 2005.

Figure 12-2: From Dudek RW, Fix JD. *Board Review Series: Embryology*. 3rd Ed. Philadelphia: Lippincott Williams & Wilkins, 2005.

Figure 12-3: From Dudek RW, Fix JD. *Board Review Series: Embryology*. 3rd Ed. Philadelphia: Lippincott Williams & Wilkins, 2005.

Figure 12-4: From Sadler TW. *Langman's Medical Embryology*. 9th Ed. Philadelphia: Lippincott Williams & Wilkins, 2004:391–393.

Figure 12-5: From McMillan JA, DeAngelis CD, Feigin RD, et al., eds. *Oski's Pediatrics: Principles and Practice*. 3rd Ed. Philadelphia: Lippincott Williams & Wilkins, 1999:394.

Figure 12-6: From Kirks DR, Griscom NT. *Practical Pediatric Imaging*. 3rd Ed. Philadelphia: Lippincott Williams & Wilkins, 1998:245.

Figure 12-7: Courtesy of Dr. A. Shaw, Department of Surgery, University of Virginia.

Figure 12-9: From Fletcher MA. *Physical Diagnosis in Neonatology*. Philadelphia: Lippincott-Raven, 1998:225. From Kirks DR, Griscom NT. *Practical Pediatric Imaging*. 3rd Ed. Philadelphia: Lippincott Williams & Wilkins, 1998:246.

Figure 12-10: From Bickley LS, Szilagyi P. *Bates' Guide to Physical Examination and History Taking*. 8th Ed. Philadelphia: Lippincott Williams & Wilkins, 2003.

Figure 12-11: From Sadler TW. *Langman's Medical Embryology*. 9th Ed. Philadelphia: Lippincott Williams & Wilkins, 2004:395. Courtesy of Dr. M. Edgerton, Department of Plastic Surgery, University of Virginia.

Figure 13-1: Modified from Truex RC, Carpenter MB. *Human Neuroanatomy*. Baltimore: Williams & Wilkins, 1969:91.

Figure 13-2: Modified from Johnson KE. *NMS Human Developmental Anatomy*. Baltimore: Williams & Wilkins, 1988:177.

Figure 13-3: From Sadler TW. *Langman's Medical Embryology*. 9th Ed. Philadelphia: Lippincott Williams & Wilkins, 2004:445.

Figure 13-4: Modified from Sadler TW. *Langman's Medical Embryology*. 6th Ed. Baltimore: Williams & Wilkins, 1990:373.

Figure 13-5: From Sadler TW. *Langman's Medical Embryology*. 9th Ed. Philadelphia: Lippincott Williams & Wilkins, 2004.

Figure 13-6: From Fletcher MA. *Physical Diagnosis in Neonatology*. Philadelphia: Lippincott-Raven, 1998:391.

Figure 13-7: Courtesy of Dr. M. J. Sellers, Division of Medical and Molecular Genetics, Guy's Hospital, London.

Figure 13-8: From Sadler TW. *Langman's Medical Embryology*. 9th Ed. Philadelphia: Lippincott Williams & Wilkins, 2004:468.

Figure 13-9: From Fletcher MA. *Physical Diagnosis in Neonatology*. Philadelphia: Lippincott-Raven, 1998:200.

Figure 13-10: From Swischuk LE. *Imaging of the Newborn, Infant, and Young Child*. 5th Ed. Philadelphia: Lippincott Williams & Wilkins, 2004.

Figure 13-12: From Swischuk LE. *Imaging of the Newborn, Infant, and Young Child*. 5th Ed. Philadelphia: Lippincott Williams & Wilkins, 2004.

Figure 13-13: From Siegel MJ. *Pediatric Sonography*. 3rd Ed. Philadelphia: Lippincott Williams & Wilkins, 2001.

Figure 14-1: (A,B,D) From Dudek RW, Fix JD. *Board Review Series: Embryology*. 3rd Ed. Philadelphia: Lippincott Williams & Wilkins, 2005:86. (C) From Sadler TW. *Langman's Medical Embryology*. 9th Ed. Philadelphia: Lippincott Williams & Wilkins, 2004:406. (E) From Rohen JW, Yokochi C, Lutken-Drecoll E, et al. *Color Atlas of Anatomy*. 4th Ed. Philadelphia: Lippincott Williams & Wilkins, 1998:124.

Figure 14-2: From Fletcher MA. *Physical Diagnosis in Neonatology*. Philadelphia: Lippincott-Raven, 1998.

Figure 14-3: From Fletcher MA. *Physical Diagnosis in Neonatology*. Philadelphia: Lippincott-Raven, 1998.

Figure 14-4: From Fletcher MA. *Physical Diagnosis in Neonatology*. Philadelphia: Lippincott-Raven, 1998.

Figure 14-6: From Kirks DR, Griscom NT. *Practical Pediatric Imaging*. 3rd Ed. Philadelphia: Lippincott Williams & Wilkins, 1998.

Figure 15-1: Modified from Dudek RW, Fix JD. *Board Review Series: Embryology*. 3rd Ed. Philadelphia: Lippincott Williams & Wilkins, 2005:84.

Figure 15-2: From Dudek RW, Fix JD. *Board Review Series: Embryology*. 3rd Ed. Philadelphia: Lippincott Williams & Wilkins, 2005:94.

Figure 15-3: From Bergsma D. *Birth Defects: Atlas and Compendium*. Baltimore: Williams & Wilkins, 1973.

Figure 15-4: From Tasman W, Jaeger E. *The Wills Eye Hospital Atlas of Clinical Ophthalmology*. 2nd Ed. Philadelphia: Lippincott Williams & Wilkins, 2001.

Figure 15-5: From Tasman W, Jaeger E. *The Wills Eye Hospital Atlas of Clinical Ophthalmology*. 2nd Ed. Philadelphia: Lippincott Williams & Wilkins, 2001.

Figure 15-6: From Sadler TW. *Langman's Medical Embryology*. 9th Ed. Philadelphia: Lippincott Williams & Wilkins, 2003.

Figure 15-7: **Left panel.** From Kirks DR, Griscom NT. *Practical Pediatric Imaging*. 3rd Ed. Philadelphia: Lippincott Williams & Wilkins, 1998. **Right panel.** From Sternberg SS. *Diagnostic Surgical Pathology*. Vol. 1. 3rd Ed. Philadelphia: Lippincott Williams & Wilkins, 1999:993.

Figure 16-1: From Dudek RW, Fix JD. *Board Review Series: Embryology*. 3rd Ed. Philadelphia: Lippincott Williams & Wilkins, 2005:204.

Figure 16-2: **(A)** From LifeART Collection Images, copyright© 2004, Lippincott Williams & Wilkins. All rights reserved. **(B)** From Crapo JD, Glassroth J, Karlinsky JB, and King TE Jr. *Baum's Textbook of Pulmonary Diseases*. 7th Ed. Philadelphia: Lippincott Williams & Wilkins, 2004.

Figure 16-3: From Fenoglio-Preiser CM, Noffsinger AE, Stemmermann GE, et al., eds. *Gastrointestional Pathology: An Atlas and Text*. 2nd Ed. Philadelphia: Lippincott Williams & Wilkins, 1998:43.

Figure 17-1: From Costanzo LS. *Board Review Series: Physiology*. 4th Ed. Philadelphia: Lippincott Williams & Wilkins, 2007:270.

Index

A

D

E

F

I

J

K

L

M

N

O

P

Q

R

T

U

V

W

Y

Z